DECISION RESEARCH

A Field Guide

John S. Carroll
Eric J. Johnson

Applied Social Research Methods Series
Volume 22

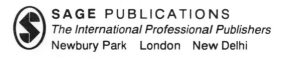
SAGE PUBLICATIONS
The International Professional Publishers
Newbury Park   London   New Delhi

For information address:

ERRATUM

Please note that the ISBNs listed on the copyri
follows:

D
C 8039 32685
P 8039 32693

Printed in the United States of America

Library of Congress Cataloging-in-Publication Data

Carroll, John S.
    Decision research : a field guide / John S. Carroll and Eric
J. Johnson
        p. cm. — (Applied social research methods series ; v. 22)
    Includes bibliographical references and index.
    ISBN 0-8039-3368-5. — ISBN 0-8039-3869-3 (pbk.)
        1. Decision-making—Research—Methodology. I. Johnson, Eric J.
II. Title. III. Series.
BF448.C37   1990
153.8′3′072—dc20   90-37006
                                                           CIP

FIRST PRINTING, 1990

Sage Production Editor: Kimberley A. Clark

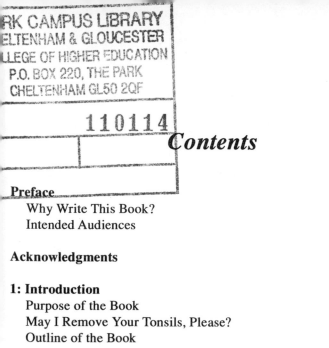

Contents

Preface

WHY WRITE THIS BOOK?

There is an ancient Chinese saying that has been paraphrased as, "If you give a starving man some fish, he can eat for a day. If you teach the man to fish, he can feed himself and his family for a lifetime."

We would like to think that a research methods book teaches the reader how to learn about decision making, instead of telling what others have discovered about the topic. Because we really believe a book about research methods in decision making is needed, we have tried to write a methods book that is interesting, knowledgeable, useful, and maybe inspiring.

INTENDED AUDIENCES

This book is ideally suited to be used in a first course on the study of decision making. Typically, there would be other books or readings that provide the theories, principles, empirical phenomena, and other substance of decision making. Readers of a book about research methods probably have orientations toward doing their own research (of an applied or theoretical nature), or possibly want to be able to appraise critically or commission research.

The prototypical student would be a first- or second-year graduate student, or an advanced undergraduate. Although decision research most typically is conducted in psychology departments, it is also appropriate for other disciplines such as political science, sociology, economics, and engineering. The most rapidly growing segments of the world of decision research are currently found in professional schools such as management, medicine, education, and public policy.

It is not necessary, however, to be a student to appreciate methods for studying decision making. Professionals who make decisions, negotiate with others, or manage other decision makers all have practical interests in decision making. These interests include particular decisions and extend to predicting and enhancing decision making in general. We believe this book can help practitioners conduct useful research or commission such research by their staff or consultants.

We have therefore written this book for a broad audience that has no special background in the subject matter of decision making, nor any high degree of expertise in behavioral research. We do assume, however, that the reader already is familiar with traditional behavioral research methods such as questionnaires, interviews, and experiments.

ACKNOWLEDGMENTS

It is important to recognize the contributions of our colleagues and friends to this book. Len Bickman, as Series Editor, was the person who first envisioned this book and kept pushing us to do it. John Payne, Jim Shanteau, Max Bazerman, Gary McClelland, and Debra Rog have made innumerable suggestions that we have tried to incorporate. Students in the Marketing Seminar at Carnegie-Mellon University read an earlier draft and were generous with their comments. Finally, without the support and consideration of Helaine Carroll, Mike Carroll, Deb Carroll, and Deborah Mitchell, this book would have been impossible.

We would also like to acknowledge the agencies whose grants and contracts supported us during the time that this book was written. John Carroll was supported by Grant SES-8510484 from the Decision, Risk, and Management Science Program of the National Science Foundation and by Grant SES-8719659 from the Law and Social Sciences Program of the National Science Foundation. Eric Johnson was supported by a grant from the Engineering Psychology program at the Office of Naval Research and by Grants SES-8809299 and SES-8721123 from the Decision, Risk, and Management Science Program of the National Science Foundation.

1

Introduction

PURPOSE OF THE BOOK

The past thirty years have ushered in a "cognitive revolution" in the social and brain sciences (National Research Council, 1982). The information-processing approach to human behavior has emerged as a mature alternative to stimulus-response and psychodynamic views. This approach presents people as purposive, reasoning "problem solvers," neither blindly seeking pleasure nor driven by inner passions, but making their own decisions in a complex and challenging world.

The theme of decision making has proven valuable in a wide range of contexts. Although most of the empirical research has involved individual choice, decision behavior has been of central interest to economists interested in the behavior of markets and economies, political scientists studying policymakers and voters, social psychologists studying groups, and organizational theorists studying the management of business and government agencies.

Despite the importance of the study of decision making, we lack textbooks about the substance and methods of decision research. Individual seminal scholars have developed particular approaches and taught them to their students in apprenticeship models. Some specific approaches have appeared in book form (Anderson, 1981; Ericsson & Simon, 1984; Keeney & Raiffa, 1976). Brief introductory books on behavioral decision theory have recently appeared (Bazerman, 1986; Dawes, 1988; Hogarth, 1987). No text, however, exists that integrates the multiple approaches that are recognized in the decision research area (Hammond, McClelland, & Mumpower, 1980, classified and reviewed six major approaches to the study of individual decision behavior; and Hammond & Arkes, 1987, have reprinted some of the classic works).

The purpose of this book is to give a concise framework for the study of decision behavior, focusing on the method rather than theories or empirical results. Both new and experienced decision researchers need to understand the range of available methods, the factors governing the appropriateness of specific methods for specific problems, and concepts underlying the ways research is conducted on decision behavior. Research and researchers—and the world they study—never stand still. To face new problems, create new methods, and combine techniques in new ways requires more than a "cookbook." We hope to provide concepts that enable good research now, and foster even better research later.

MAY I REMOVE YOUR TONSILS, PLEASE?

As a student in public school during the 1950s, the first author of this book remembers having conversations about children undergoing surgery for the removal of tonsils. There were stories about hospitals and ice cream after throat surgery, and medical "lineups" at which doctors would check kids for unhealthy tonsils. It never occurred to most students that doctors might be wrong about the usefulness of tonsillectomies (the surgical removal of tonsils), or that these diagnostic procedures might have a touch of superstitious ritual.

Before either author of this book was born, the *New England Journal of Medicine* described a research study of medical decisions regarding tonsillectomies (Bakwin, 1945). The researchers recruited a panel of three physicians to screen all 389 5th-grade schoolboys from one town. The panel recommended that 45% of the boys undergo surgical removal of their tonsils. The physicians were thanked and dismissed. A second panel of three physicians was recruited and asked to examine the 215 boys who had been judged by the first panel *not* to need surgery. If there was complete agreement between the panels of physicians, then none of these boys should have been judged to need tonsillectomies; in fact, 46% were judged to need surgery. It was as if the initial screening had never occurred! Then, the second panel of physicians was dismissed and a third panel recruited to examine the 116 boys who had been twice cleared. The third panel diagnosed 44% of these boys as needing tonsillectomies.

Although the participating doctors were trying to make good decisions, and felt capable of making these decisions, the results were very disappointing. The doctors seemed to lack consistency from panel to panel. Were they choosing randomly? Probably not—the doctors would surely argue that their diagnoses were based on the physical attributes of the tonsils (size, color, etc.). It seems unlikely that the doctors on the three panels were using different rules, since medical training and aggregation into panels should level out idiosyncratic decision rules.

Instead, it is possible that the doctors were making *relative* judgments about each set of tonsils in the context of other recently seen tonsils. In any set of children, the diagnostic standards may get reset as the children pass through. In this study, the successive waves of students had smaller tonsils, but doctors were insensitive to absolute size; within each set of boys, they selected the biggest and reddest tonsils for surgery.

This study illustrates why research on decision making is interesting and important. First, it is not obvious how decision makers—even experts—make decisions. Even the decision makers themselves may be mistaken about their decision behavior. Second, years of training and practice in making decisions do not necessarily perfect decision quality. Third, it may be useful to consider how decisions are made in terms of the information used, the way information is combined, the situational effects on decision making (e.g., time pressure, groups versus individuals), and the kind of feedback received about decision quality. Fourth, it may be useful to think of how to improve decision making—for example, what to tell doctors in order to avoid unnecessary tonsillectomies. Despite publication of the article discussed above in one of the best journals of medical research, it took many years for tonsillectomies to fall from acceptable medical wisdom. Could we help doctors make better decisions, for example, by providing an explicit decision rule including a standard picture chart of tonsils to compare visually against every patient?

OUTLINE OF THE BOOK

This chapter provides a rationale for the book and a map for the topics to be presented, as well as a set of criteria on which to judge research methods. The intention is to have a consistent viewpoint from which to evaluate each of the diverse group of techniques that are used in studying decision making. Finally, suggestions are offered for developing research questions—the starting point for any use of research methods.

Chapter 2 presents a brief introduction to the field of decision making. It is intended for readers who do not have any facility with the concepts and principles of the field; those with prior background are encouraged to skip the chapter or skim through. In Chapter 2, we offer some arguments for why decision making is an important topic for study, and establish definitions of major concepts to be used throughout the book. The chapter includes a brief summary of some substantive findings from the field of decision making, to orient the reader and to exemplify the process of formulating research questions.

In Chapter 3, we discuss the most typical and least formal methods of studying decision making. We are all comfortable with simply asking people to report about past decisions; continuing our example of medical decision making, one could ask doctors how they decide about tonsillectomies. We treat this as a serious method, explore the pros and cons of self-reporting, and suggest some reasons why this informal method is necessary yet problematic. We will also examine case methods that use a variety of observational techniques to reach an understanding of particular decisions or decision makers—for example, directly observing one or a few doctors screening children for unhealthy tonsils.

In Chapter 4, we discuss a series of methods that investigate decision making through observation and measurement in naturalistic settings. These methods produce what we call *weighted additive models* that relate mathematical combinations of the attribute information available to the decision maker to the decision maker's judgments or choices. In the case of medical diagnosis, we might obtain or create a set of actual diagnostic decisions, including information about the size and redness of tonsils, ages of patients, and other features of each case. From these data, we could build a model of how the doctors decide about tonsillectomies.

Chapter 5 extends our concepts of decision making by exploring in more detail the processes by which decision makers collect and assemble information, use various strategies to combine information and make inferences, and produce judgments or decisions. A series of methods called *process-tracing techniques* are described whose purpose is to observe mental processes as closely as possible during decision making. In this manner, for example, one might ask doctors to "think aloud," talking about each case as they examine each child's tonsils.

Chapter 6 introduces methods that impose more artificial controls on decision situations. These methods can be used for the development of theories of decision making as well as the study of particular decisions. These include highly stylized decision situations in which information and objectives are experimentally manipulated by the researchers, and various hypothetical questions directed at particular features of the way people make decisions. One could, for example, create artificial sets of cases for doctors to diagnose, including different photographs of tonsils and case sets with different distributions of tonsil size and redness.

Chapter 7 examines the practical problems involved in carrying out a decision research project. Not everyone wishes to have their decisions examined; there are important issues of access, confidentiality, the use of research, and ethics that must be considered in any research project. Surely, doctors who are told that their decisions are inconsistent, or that they are recommending unnecessary surgery, would be very upset. It is hoped that they would take a positive view—that this is a way to improve medical practice—rather than a negative view that the researchers are furthering their careers by destroying doctors.

Finally, in Chapter 8 we take a look back at all the research methods to assess their strengths and weaknesses, then look at what the future of decision research might hold. The field of decision research is only about thirty years old. In this short time, theories, empirical results, and methods have changed dramatically. It will continue to be a vibrant area of study.

There is a Chinese saying, "May you live in interesting times," that is used as both a blessing and a curse. We believe that the current development of decision research makes our times very interesting. For the researcher, this is a blessing; but there is much to be done.

EVALUATING DECISION RESEARCH METHODS

There are many possible criteria that could be assembled for evaluating the methods we will present in this book. We could talk about advancing science, generalizability, useful applications, and so forth. We have chosen to focus on six criteria of the benefits and costs of decision research:

1. *Discovery*—having the power to uncover new phenomena, surprise the researcher, and lead to creative insights.

2. *Understanding*—providing a cause-and-effect analysis that uncovers the mechanisms or processes by which decisions are made.

3. *Prediction*—having logical or mathematical rules that predict the judgment and decisions that will be made. These rules need not represent the actual decision processes.

4. *Prescriptive Control*—providing opportunities and techniques for changing the decision process, as in prescribing better decision rules or testing potential manipulations.

5. *Confound Control*—creating controlled situations so as to rule out other explanations of the results (known as *confounds*).

6. *Ease of Use*—taking less time and resources for the same progress toward the other goals.

As each research method is presented and discussed, we will use the above criteria to assess its advantages and disadvantages, as somewhat of a "consumer's guide" to research. By the concluding chapter, we will be able to compare and contrast the major classes of methods and their appropriateness for various situations.

RESEARCH QUESTIONS

Perhaps the most difficult part of conducting good research is thinking of good research questions. Training programs tend to be very good at teaching specific research methods and analytical skills for criticizing research, but rarely direct attention at the process of defining research projects in the first place (for some general insights, see Daft, 1984; Lundberg, 1976; Martin, 1982).

We have a few suggestions for generic research questions about decision making, or heuristics for the generation of such research questions. We do this by proposing three dimensions along which research questions might vary: the unit, the goal, and the stage.

The Unit: Which Decisions and Decision Makers Are of Interest?

Research may be conducted to examine a particular decision, a particular kind of decision, a particular decision maker, or aspects of the decision process in general. The study of a particular decision would involve seeking to understand just one event. Historians might wish to know why and how Abraham Lincoln decided to free the slaves; the Coca-Cola company might want to analyze how it went wrong in replacing the old Coke with the new Coke; a parent might want to know why her child was diagnosed as needing surgery. If, instead, we wish to study a particular kind of decision, then we must look at many events that share a common content. For example, how do judges determine sentences? How to weather experts predict the weather? How do stock analysts pick stocks? And how do doctors diagnose tonsils?

Focusing on particular decision makers might lead us to study the Warren Supreme Court, to classify managers as analytical or intuitive, or to study older doctors versus younger doctors. Finally, studying aspects of the decision process leads to questions that decompose decisions into stages and processes: what choice rules do decision makers use, and under what circumstances? How does past experience with decisions affect problem formulation? How does feedback improve decision making?

The Goal: What Do We Hope to Achieve?

Research can be directed at several different goals. Traditionally, we think in terms of understanding, prediction, and control. Research questions directed at understanding decision making would be directed toward the mechanisms and causes of various decision behaviors. How do personal, contextual, and task attributes combine to influence the decision? Why do decision makers attend to particular information, rely on certain sources, or set particular goals? Why are particular strategies used to put information together? How was a specific decision made?

Research questions directed at prediction need to put together the various elements that influence decision making into a predictive model, but that model need not work in the same way that the decision makers do (Hoffman, 1960). If we simply predict, for example, that people will decide by habit, or follow their single most important criterion, we would be right quite often without needing to understand why we were right. Many financiers would be very happy to be able to predict business cycles, regardless of whether their theories offered an adequate understanding of the underlying processes.

Finally, research questions oriented toward control generally seek to improve decision making. What kinds of decision aids—such as expert systems, decision support systems, or simple checklists—are most helpful? What decisions should be assigned to groups, rather than individuals? Should we increase or decrease the role of intuition in decision making?

The Stages of Decision Making:
Analyzing the Components

Decision researchers assume that decision making occurs in a series of fairly well-defined stages, although a particular decision could repeat and backtrack in a complex way. Distilling the comments of several theorists (Einhorn & Hogarth, 1981; Engel, Blackwell, & Miniard, 1986; Huber, 1980), we can produce the following list of stages: (1) recognition; (2) formulation; (3) alternative generation; (4) information search; (5) judgment or choice; (6) action; and (7) feedback. Although common sense defines decision making as information search and choice—and theorists sometimes distinguish this narrow view of decision making from the broader process of "problem solving" (Huber, 1980)—we will take the broad view that the study of decision making is concerned with all of the above stages. These stages, and the basic components and processes of decision making, are more fully discussed in Chapter 2.

Table 1.1

Typical Research Questions for Each Decision Stage

Recognition	Who noticed the problem? What had to happen in order for this to be labeled as a decision problem?
Formulation	Who defined the problem? How could it be separated or combined with other problems? Did different people define it differently? What goals emerged and whose goals are they?
Alternative Generation	Where did the alternatives come from? How was it decided to stop generating alternatives?
Information Search	How much information was collected about each alternative? Was the same information collected about each? Was the search confirmatory of an already preferred alternative?
Evaluation/Choice	What kind of judgments were made? By whom? What kinds of knowledge were used to turn information into meaningful categories and dimensions? What assumptions were made in order to apply the rules?
Action/Feedback	What happened after the decision? Did the decision have to be justified, and to whom?

Using this sequence of decision stages, Table 1.1 lists some generic research questions that typically are considered important to decision researchers. (The table should only be considered illustrative or provocative, rather than exhaustive.)

By using the three dimensions of unit, goal, and stage, readers of this book should be able to generate some research questions of their own, which can then be addressed using the methods that are presented in the following chapters.

SKILL BUILDING

Those with less background in decision making may find it beneficial to read Chapter 2 (which provides an introduction to the concepts and research results of the field of decision making) before tackling these exercises.

1. Consider the last time you made a major consumer purchase, such as a car, stereo system, camera, house, or washing machine.

   (a) Describe each stage of your decision. What were your goals, your alternatives, the attributes you considered, your sources of information, and the strategies you used? What were the outcomes, and did you learn anything to help you make decisions in the future?

   (b) Who would be interested in knowing how you decided? You? Your spouse? Your boss? Marketers or decision scientists? Why would they be interested, and what goals could they achieve?

   (c) Formulate one question that you would like to have answered about that decision. What sort of research question is it, in terms of unit, goal, and stage?

2. Consider the last presidential election. Of what value would it have been to various people to *understand* why the election turned out as it did? Who would have wanted to be able to *predict* the outcome, and why? Who would find it useful to *control* or influence voting, and why?

3. List two or three research questions that are of interest to you right now. What is it about these questions that makes them interesting to you? What would you do or think differently if you knew the answers to these questions?

2

A Primer on Decision Making

THE DECISION-MAKING PERSPECTIVE

Decision making is a process by which a person, group, or organization identifies a choice or judgment to be made, gathers and evaluates information about alternatives, and selects from among the alternatives. For example, consider what happens when a patient comes to a doctor with various complaints and symptoms (e.g., Elstein & Bordage, 1979). Through a process of information gathering that relates the current situation to the doctor's experience and training, the doctor decides that the patient most likely has a bacterial infection (a diagnosis of the *problem*). The doctor then prescribes a drug regimen that is effective against a wide variety of bacteria (a choice among *actions*). Subsequently, the patient decides whether or not to follow the regimen (patients often stop when they feel good, which may be too soon), and the doctor may have to reevaluate the situation if the patient does not improve.

The usefulness of this approach rests solely on its ability to provide explanations and insights that are novel, integrative, and applicable. The same is true for any approach. It is our belief that the decision-making approach has demonstrated its value and continues to offer exciting new knowledge.

THE VALUE OF DECISION RESEARCH

If decision making were easy to understand (or easy to do), there would be no need for elaborate research efforts. As illustrated in Chapter 1 regarding medical diagnoses, however, research consistently reveals that decision makers often diverge from what is considered desirable behavior, and show less insight into their own behavior than might be guessed. Gradually, we are learning that decision making in a broad range of domains (e.g., medicine, business, law) is flawed but subject to improvement if we understand the decision task and the decision makers.

To illustrate the generality of decision research, let us take a second example from a different domain: finance. Decision researchers have been studying stock portfolio selection for many years (Ebert & Kruse, 1978; Slovic, 1969) and have drawn some interesting conclusions that contradict common sense and expert wisdom. First, although portfolio managers claim to use a large number of information cues or factors in selecting stock investments, their decisions can be imitated quite well by models containing only a few cues or pieces of information. Second, novices do about as well as experts in picking stocks. Third, the experts fall prey to the same common-sense errors as do the novices. Fourth, simple statistical prediction models outperform the experts. Finally, models based on the experts' own simple rules outperform the experts themselves, indicating that the experts are inconsistent in applying what they know (rules and relationships) to apparently unique instances and are easily overloaded by information.

The managerial payoff for knowledge such as this is to enable a restructuring of the decision situation. A company called Batterymarch in Boston developed its own strikingly parallel understanding of what decision makers do well and what they do poorly, and used it to restructure its stock portfolio management. In the Batterymarch system, the expert analyst seeks to uncover new rules or principles that are then tested using computerized data bases of past stock performance. Useful and proven rules are incorporated into a computer program that makes portfolio decisions about classes of stocks. Individual analysts do not make buy/sell decisions about individual stocks for accounts; these are all made by computer. Thus, the experts do exactly what people are best at: seeing new patterns and testing creative ideas. The computer does exactly what people are worst at: manipulating large amounts of data and applying rules to specific decision situations in a consistent manner.

No decision process, however, is without risk: the stock market crash of 1987 was exacerbated by computerized trading routines that moved large blocks of stock so rapidly that no one realized the special nature of the circumstances and the need to reconsider the use and design of automated routines.

THE NATURE OF DECISION MAKING

It is not easy to break up a stream of thoughts and behaviors into units called "decisions." For example, shoppers can be thought of as deciding what brand of coffee to buy. Yet they may also be deciding *how* to decide, in the sense of which brands to consider, what information to gather, how to weight various issues (price, bitterness, aroma), and what decision rules to use (see Humphreys & Berkeley, 1983). There may not even be an explicit decision if all they do is to implement a previous "standing decision" to buy their regular brand, without considering any alternatives. The concept of a decision is really a shorthand for mental activities that recognize and structure decision situations and then evaluate preferences to produce judgments and choices (Kahneman & Tversky, 1979; Einhorn & Hogarth, 1981).

To cut through this complexity we need a consistent and coherent map of the temporal stages of decision making, and the components and dimensions of decision making.

Temporal Stages of Decision Making

As mentioned in Chapter 1, decision making may be outlined in a series of fairly well-defined stages. These stages are: (1) recognition; (2) formulation; (3) alternative generation; (4) information search; (5) judgment or choice; (6) action; and (7) feedback. The following sections explore these stages and discuss key concepts that are the building blocks of theory and research.

Recognition. The process of decision making begins with the realization that there is a decision to make. Many activities that are not "decisions" per se but are relevant to decisions occur prior to recognition or result in recognition. Nonspecific information search activity, such as reading a newspaper or talking about cars with friends, could be considered as "predecisional" activity (see Payne, Braunstein, & Carroll, 1978) undertaken to prepare for future (unspecified) decisions. Thus, almost all behavior is potentially relevant to present and future decisions. When people avoid defining a particular situation as a "decision" or deliberately avoid making decisions (e.g., Corbin, 1980; Isenberg, 1984), this is also a predecisional act.

Formulation. When a situation is recognized as a decision problem, the next stage involves exploring and classifying the decision situation, including some understanding of relevant objectives and values. The decision making perspective assumes that people try to achieve preferred outcomes, objectives, or goals, even though they may be unsure, in error, or unable to express their concepts of value. In shopping for a car, for example, a customer may have concerns or preferences regarding price, appearance, size, handling, and economy. In addition, there may be concerns regarding the decision process, such as minimizing time and avoiding high-pressure salespeople.

Alternative generation. Even the simple act of buying breakfast cereal could be viewed as a complex mental feat of choosing among all possible combinations of cereals offered in a typical store. Although this is theoretically true, actual decision makers do not consider all these alternatives, instead structuring the decision as something like "pick two of my usual four cereals," or "replace what has been eaten." Through prior habits, exposure to advertising, or the arrangement of shelf space, the number of alternatives that attract attention—the "consideration set" (Bettman, 1979)—is tremendously reduced.

An employer seeking to hire two employees first must seek out possible candidates through job notices, word of mouth, and so forth. If satisfactory candidates do not surface easily, more intensive procedures (such as the use of a headhunter) are tried. Even after a decision is "made," the employer may stumble across a new prospect that leads to a reevaluation. Notice that the best decision rule in this case might not be to hire the top two all-around candidates, but rather to look for more diversity of skills: Choosing two employees out of ten possibilities could be structured as choosing from among 45 possible pairs of employees!

Information search. In order to make a sensible decision, decision makers seek to identify the attributes or properties of the alternatives under consideration. When a shopper chooses a breakfast cereal to buy in the grocery store, the shopper can read the attributes on the cereal box, knows its price, and (for familiar cereals) also knows the outcomes he or she will get when consuming the cereal. We call such a situation in which the alternatives have known outcomes *decision under certainty* or *riskless choice*.

Someone considering buying a state lottery ticket, however, does not know what the outcome will be, but does know (or could easily find out) the likelihood of winning various amounts. This situation is similar to a bet over a coin flip, where there is a 50-50 chance of winning or losing some money; the attributes of the alternatives (bet, or don't bet) are amounts of money and likelihood or probability, and they are known. This situation is called *decision under uncertainty* or *risky choice*.

Now consider a female sales manager who is trying to hire a salesman. During the employment interview, she finds out that the candidate grew up in her neighborhood. From the written application, she reads that the candidate has an impressive past record of sales experience and effectiveness. During their conversation, the candidate is alert, makes eye contact, and laughs at the manager's jokes. From this information, we can make predictions of the candidate's future performance, but the probability of any outcome is hard to divine. This situation (in which the uncertainties are themselves unspecified) is called *decision under ambiguity.* Ambiguity increases the difficulty of identifying the "best" decision.

Judgment or choice. Judgment and choice are really two different kinds of decision making that can, at times, produce different decisions (Abelson & Levi, 1985; Tversky, Sattath, & Slovic, 1988). We will find that different research methods are appropriate for these different decision tasks.

In a judgment task, one places a label on a single alternative or attribute. A judgment task can be thought of as a kind of comparison or matching task, in the sense that an alternative or attribute is matched to a response scale label. In the above scenario, the manager may characterize the job candidate as similar to herself, good at selling, and socially adept or smooth. Such subjective judgments are themselves like higher order attributes of the salesperson. Other examples are easy to find. When *Consumer Reports* evaluates cars on five-point scales for safety and handling, it is judging alternatives (cars) on attributes. By rating the "importance" of various aspects of food such as taste, calories, fat content, appearance, and price, you are judging the importance of the *attributes,* themselves.

Choice involves comparisons among alternatives. The careful car buyer evaluates many attributes about many cars, and puts together this information through a complex process involving many different values and judgments; the casual buyer may quickly rule out cars on the basis of price and brand and pick the first acceptable car.

The way in which a decision maker sorts through and evaluates attributes and alternatives—for judgment or choice—is by employing *decision rules* which vary in their generality, formality, and complexity. General rules can be applied across a broad variety of decision situations. An example of a general choice rule is, "Don't change a winning strategy." Specific rules are those with a narrow range of applicability, such as "Try the hot and sour soup at any new Chinese restaurant." Formal rules have more exact specifications, often have quantitative forms, and often derive from normative theories of good decision making; informal rules tend to be more qualitative and inexact, resembling *heuristics* or rules of thumb. Complex rules have more components than simple rules, and tend therefore to require more effort (Johnson & Payne, 1985).

It is assumed that everyone has a repertoire of decision rules (Payne et al., 1978; Svenson, 1979) developed through experience and training. Therefore, we must also have higher order rules for determining when to use various rules. For example, Beach and Mitchell (1978) suggest that decision rules are chosen to balance the beneficial quality of making better choices against the costs of using more complex but better decision rules. Johnson and Payne (1985) have written an interesting analysis examining the trade-offs in using various decision rules.

Action. Once a decision is "made" in one's mind, it still must be acted upon. The recent terminology of "decision taking" seems to capture the sequence of first making a decision and then acting on it. For example, a car buyer may decide to buy a car and wake up the next day unwilling to carry out the decision. Or, events may intervene to prevent the action: the car dealer closes, the car is unavailable, credit cannot be obtained, and so forth.

Feedback. After decisions have been acted upon, the decision maker may receive information about the outcomes of the action. This permits learning—that is, changes in substantive knowledge and decision rules. We also get feedback when we justify our decisions to others, even when our justifications are untrue (Nisbett & Ross, 1980; Staw, 1980).

Medical diagnoses are an excellent example of *dynamic decision making* (Kleinmuntz, 1985), in which a series of related decisions and actions provide information over time that enables the decision maker to spread the decision process out over time. By choosing various tests, and choosing treatments that produce feedback, a doctor narrows in on an effective diagnosis and treatment (or a treatment that works without full understanding). Researchers recently have recognized the importance of dynamic tasks in contrast to static or "one-shot" laboratory tasks (Connolly, 1982; Hogarth, 1981; Sterman, 1989).

An Example: Jury Decisions

A good example of how decisions can be examined in temporal stages is jury decision making. This is an interesting situation in part because different stages are assigned to different people. Jurors are selected on the basis of having *no* prior knowledge of a case or defendant. Thus objectivity is essentially equated with no meaningful predecisional activity prior to the trial. Information gathering is exclusively the responsibility of the attorneys on both sides. They present attributes and judgments, and suggest appropriate decisions, but the power of making the decision (that is, of choosing to say "guilty" or "innocent") rests with the jury. During the trial, the judge has the role of monitoring the decision procedures for fairness and keeping everyone within the rules. After the trial is over, there is no formal feedback to jurors; the only feedback is through the media and what their friends and family say to them. They rarely find out that they were "right" or "wrong."

How Do People Decide?

In order to create new and useful research, or to apply decision research methods to a specific situation, it is helpful to know the kinds of results that typically emerge from the field of decision research. The following brief summary is meant to orient the reader rather than to "tell it all." To understand the theoretical and empirical bases of decision research in depth would take some reading of key books and collections of papers (e.g., Arkes & Hammond, 1986; Hogarth, 1987; Kahneman, Slovic, & Tversky, 1982).

Rational models and cognitive biases. Normative theories of decision making, such as classical economic theory (von Neumann & Morgenstern, 1944), propose that decision makers follow a highly rational procedure for making decisions. They assume that decision makers have consistent preferences, know their preferences, know the alternatives available, have access to information about the consequences of selecting each alternative, and combine the information according to the expected utility rule, which discounts or weights outcomes by their probability of occurrence (Dawes, 1988; Fischhoff, 1982).

Although these principles are logical and appealing (and based on theories that guarantee the best long-term chance for successful outcomes), research evidence shows that actual decisions consistently diverge from the rational model. For example, it is puzzling why so many people are basically honest about paying their taxes, because the likelihood of being caught is quite low and the penalty for being caught is modest (repaying the missing tax plus 50%) (Blumstein, 1983). In fact, by using the rational model as a benchmark, we can show consistent errors or biases when actual decisions are compared against the "optimal" decisions prescribed by the normative model (Bazerman, 1986; Dawes, 1988; Hogarth, 1987; Kahneman, Slovic, & Tversky, 1982).

It is important to recognize that the economic model of rationality has not been disproved by such research. Economists have argued that the normative models do not apply to situations when people don't really care about how well they do, or lack sufficient understanding of their positions. If people have the wrong information—such as believing they have a better chance of winning the lottery than is objectively true—then we should not be surprised that they appear to decide in error. Economists also argue that there are various nonmonetary values related to self-esteem, effort, or the thrill of gambling that make an expanded utility model very adequate. The point here is not to disprove the rational model, but to reveal phenomena that are important for theory and application.

Limited rationality. Thirty years of research in cognitive psychology have revealed that the human mind is limited in attention, memory, and calculation (Anderson, 1985; Newell & Simon, 1972). Our short-term memory for what is going on around us can hold only a few "chunks" of information at one time, and moving that information into permanent, long-term storage is difficult. For example, although you may use a telephone many times a day, and have looked at the keypad thousands of times in your life, you probably cannot reproduce the correct arrangement of letters with the numbers because there is no reason to pay attention to the letters. How much of what you did yesterday can you recall (in detail) and how much of that "memory" is really a distorted reconstruction? Furthermore, it is hard to keep several things in mind at once, making complex judgments and mental arithmetic almost impossible. Arithmetic is easy to do with pencil and paper because we need not rely on our short-term memory to hold partial calculations, call up formulas, and remember what to do next.

The effects of these limitations on judgment and decision making are quite important. Because we cannot deal with large amounts of information at one time, we tend to simplify situations, to formulate decisions through limited viewpoints that highlight some aspects of the situation but ignore others. We also have developed a great variety of shortcuts, rules of thumb, or heuristics for making reasonably good decisions within our constraints or limitations.

It's how you see the problem. People respond to situations as they interpret them, not as they exist in some objective reality. Psychologists talk about the *frame* that people use to identify decision problems and their components (Tversky & Kahneman, 1981); the same problem in a different frame can elicit a very different response. For example, most people seem more concerned about avoiding losses than achieving gains. The same situation, however, can be defined as a loss avoided or a gain achieved. Credit card companies fought hard to have only one price for consumer goods, regardless of whether they were purchased by credit card or cash. When the practice of having two prices became legal, the same companies fought to have a credit card *price* and a cash *discount*, rather than a cash *price* and a credit card *surcharge* (Thaler, 1980). A discount is a gain, whereas a surcharge is a loss. People would be more willing—in the credit card companies' view—to use the credit card when they are foregoing a gain (in comparison to the cash price) than when they are taking a loss, even though the final dollar costs are identical.

Heuristics or strategies for decision making. The study of heuristics for judgment and decision making has produced some very interesting examples of general-purpose heuristics. Consider, for example, the heuristic called *anchoring and adjustment*. To estimate an unknown such as the time it takes to write a book, an aspiring author might start with something that is known, such as the time it takes to write a page. This known element is called an anchor. A book of 200 pages could then be estimated to take 200 times as long as one page, an adjustment from the anchor. This is a reasonable approach but research evidence shows that use of anchoring-and-adjustment typically results in estimates too close to the anchor (Tversky & Kahneman, 1974). There are also innumerable examples of special-purpose heuristics that apply to particular domains such as chess (avoid trades where you lose more valuable pieces than your opponent) and consumer purchases (judge quality by price).

The key feature of heuristics is that they *usually* do a good job, but not necessarily the best job given the information at hand (and they sometimes do poorly). They are also easier for an unaided decision maker to employ than highly sophisticated decision rules such as those proposed by economists and management scientists.

Trade-offs are hard to make. Heuristics are valuable because they save effort and facilitate decisions within the constraints of cognitive limitations. They have a second function as well: they allow decision makers to avoid difficult trade-offs. For example, you may wish to buy a car that is high quality, fun to drive, and inexpensive. Unfortunately, better cars are more costly, and somehow you have to determine how much it is worth to have a little more fun or a little higher quality. It is hard to put a price on such things, so most people adopt a decision rule that does not require trading off incommensurables. For example, you may set a maximum price (what you can "afford") and then look for the most attractive option in your price range (Tversky, 1972). By ruling out all cars over the limit, you greatly simplify the decision problem and avoid putting a price on attributes that are hard to assess. Of course, you may miss the perfect car that happens to be $50 over your limit!

We are not very self-aware. Although people strive to make good decisions and often have high opinions of their own decision making, research repeatedly shows that decision makers may not understand their own implicit decision rules (Hammond, Stewart, Brehmer, & Steinmann, 1975) and are systematically overconfident about the quality of their judgments and decisions (Fischhoff, 1975).

Learning comes slowly, if at all. With experience, shouldn't we become better decision makers? The answer, of course, is yes. We get better slowly, however, and more slowly than we might hope. Studies of expert decision makers suggest that they sometimes do little (if any) better than novices, and that people sometimes learn the wrong things from "experience." Because of incomplete feedback, delayed feedback, and uncertainty—sometimes good decisions produce bad results, and vice-versa—learning from experience is much more difficult than we realize (Einhorn, 1980).

People seem quite able to "learn" all sorts of superstitious and incorrect decision rules, and to have a very difficult time unlearning them. Dice players continue to blow on the dice to encourage the right numbers to come up, analysts continue to look for patterns in the stock market that can be shown to have no relationship to future stock movements, doctors perform tonsillectomies for decades after research shows them to be unnecessary, and sports enthusiasts continue to believe in the "hot hand" in basketball (Gilovich, Vallone, & Tversky, 1985). Disconfirming instances are easily forgotten or explained away; confirming instances are remembered much more vividly.

Groups are no better. Even though individuals are flawed decision makers, will organizations or markets composed of multiple decision makers achieve a higher level of rationality? Studies that have directly compared groups and individuals on the same problems find that groups fall prey to the same errors and biases as do individuals (e.g., Argote, Seabright, & Dyer, 1986; Bazerman, Giuliano, & Appelman, 1984). Furthermore, groups have their own characteristic problems, such as a premature tendency to reach consensus (groupthink; Janis, 1982), a tendency to become even more extreme over issues where the group has an initial leaning (group polarization; Lamb & Myers, 1978), and a pervasive ability to eat up time and resources. Similarly, dyadic negotiators and markets of buyers and sellers also exhibit dysfunctions that arise from individual cognitive limitations (Bazerman, Mannix, Sondak, & Thompson, 1990).

Where groups are useful is in combining bits of information that are not held by any individual, and in providing sheer capacity for work (Steiner, 1972). Groups do not always recognize right answers when they see them, however, or identify experts in their midst (Laughlin & Ellis, 1986). Thus, there is no guarantee that a group will produce a high-quality decision even when knowledge and competency are adequate in the group as a whole.

Early in the history of information-processing approaches to problem solving and decision making, seminal efforts were made to understand groups (Davis, 1973; Hoffman, 1979) and organizations (Cyert & March, 1963; March & Simon, 1958; Simon, 1976). As March and Shapira (1982) state,

Students of cognition are understandably uncomfortable with discussions of the "cognitive behavior" of institutions. It seems natural to impute thinking, consciousness, and intentionality to individuals, somewhat less natural to use the same metaphors with regard to complex combinations of individuals. (p. 97)

It is possible to conceptualize and to study groups as collections of information processors who have varied goals, varied roles, and who communicate information in real time. Although this approach has all of the difficulties of studying individuals compounded by the complexities of the aggregation of people, efforts are being made to deepen our research on small groups (Hastie, Penrod, & Pennington, 1983; Stasser, 1988; Vinokur & Burnstein, 1974) and to develop approaches to organizational decision making (March & Shapira, 1982; Mintzberg, Raisinghani, & Theoret, 1976). Throughout this book, we will give examples of research methods in use with groups and organizations, as well as with individual decision makers.

Helping Decision Makers

Because individuals and groups are prone to error, behave inconsistently, and may not realize when their decisions are of better or worse quality, they could use some help. Most generally, the prescriptions of accountants, economists, operations researchers, and even theologians can be seen as suggestions for generally useful frames and decision rules.

Indeed, entire fields such as decision analysis (Keeney & Raiffa, 1976; von Winterfeldt & Edwards, 1986) have arisen for the purpose of helping people measure their own preferences and judgments and follow explicit procedures and rules so as to make better decisions. Interestingly, the value of decision analysis arises not simply from telling decision makers what to do, but also from the self-knowledge that is obtained through the process of analyzing problems and checking intuitions against formal rules. Similarly, decision support systems, expert systems, and artificial intelligence applications are ways to capture the knowledge of experts and either assist them in making better decisions or replace them with automated decision systems (see Chapter 8).

This brief—and, it is hoped, tantalizing—summary of some of the substantive research and theorizing about decision making should have prepared you to hear how decision researchers go about studying decision making. You can adopt the decision perspective, see people around you making judgments and decisions, and use the information in the rest of this book to find out more about what decision makers are doing. The payoffs are increased understanding of decision behavior, a better ability to predict decisions, and a chance to improve the decisions that are made by yourself and by others.

3

Asking About Decision Making

INTRODUCTION

When one of the authors of this book began what turned into a ten-year-long project on parole decisions (Carroll, Wiener, Coates, Galegher, & Alibrio, 1982), an initial set of research activities was to meet with parole decision makers, watch them make some decisions (by observing interviews in prisons), and ask them how their decisions were made. Many researchers have found that asking such simple questions is very useful, and yet the answers cannot be accepted at face value. To continue the example, the parole decision makers tended to say that they made their decisions through "intuition," "experience," "by looking at all the information in the case," and by recognizing that "every case is unique."

Decision makers frequently are unable to articulate their underlying decision processes, or are more interested in presenting a favorable impression. As a result, we need some ways to check on the accuracy and completeness of self-reports. Case methods have been developed into intensive and disciplined forms by clinical psychologists, historians, journalists, and anthropologists.

Both self-reports and case methods represent *natural* or *implicit* methods because they have everyday, commonsensical origins and uses. They are typically qualitative, rather than quantitative, in the way data are collected and interpreted. Self-reports and case methods can also be used in conjunction with the more quantitative and formal methods (to be presented in subsequent chapters) as ways to explore decision domains, generate hypotheses, and check research results.

In this chapter, we will take these methods very seriously as ways of understanding decisions and of stimulating theory development. We will express our reservations about the methods, but explain the circumstances under which such methods will and should be used.

THE SELF-REPORT METHOD

Imagine that you have called up your stockbroker to find out why she sold 200 shares of Ford and bought 100 shares of IBM on your behalf. She replies, "I used my professional judgment to get you the best results." This is probably the kind of reassuring reply that ends most such conversations. You ask, however, for a more detailed explanation. She then responds with a discussion of rate of return, risk, industry trends, price/earnings and debt/equity ratios, and so forth. You thank her for her explanation, and feel somewhat satisfied and perhaps somewhat confused.

The stockbroker first tried to give an *acceptable explanation* under the assumption that you needed reassurance that your account was receiving high quality care, rather than a technical explanation. Most people want to know that their stockbroker, doctor, or auto mechanic is "expert" or "well-recommended" without attempting to understand how their "agent" makes decisions (see Petty & Cacioppo, 1981).

When you rejected her initial response, the stockbroker shifted to a more technical discussion of what constitutes "good results"—providing an informal model of her decision process using the same components that we will see in more formal methods: (1) goals or objectives; (2) sources of information about the expected consequences of possible alternatives; and (3) procedures or rules for generating a decision from the goals and information. It is important, however, to consider whether she was reporting on decisions as they are being made, as they were recently made, as they were made some time ago, as they will be made, or as they are generally made.

As a second example, Henry Ford, founder of the Ford Motor Company dynasty, told *The Detroit News*,

> It is better to sell a large number of cars at a reasonably small margin than to sell fewer cars at a large margin of profit. . . . It enables a larger number of people to buy and enjoy [the car] and it gives a larger number of men employment at good wages. Those are two aims I have in life. (Lacey, 1986, p. 169)

This statement is a retrospective account of the values and decision rules underlying a large set of operational decisions. It would be a useful answer to questions such as, "Why did you lower the price of the Model T to $400?" Notice, however, that saying you are in business to make consumers and workers happy will probably make the audience like you (and buy your cars). Because the degree to which such self-reports are *true* is so central to the usefulness of the methods, we will first discuss the problems with self-reporting before providing details of how to use the method.

Problems With Self-Reports

The overall goal of studying decisions is to produce useful information. In order to be useful, the information we obtain must be relevant to our needs, sufficiently detailed or precise, reliable, and valid. In the terminology of Chris Argyris (1976; Argyris & Schon, 1974), we must distinguish *espoused theories* consisting of the goals, assumptions, and values that people claim guide their decisions from *theories-in-use* that are the actual guides to decisions.

In the examples of the stockbroker and Henry Ford, it is easy to identify some threats to the usefulness of the responses: (1) In the process of *remembering* what they did in any specific instance, they may have forgotten parts of the decision; (2) they may be *reconstructing* the decision process by using what they usually do or what they are supposed to do, rather than reporting what they actually did; and (3) they may be *rationalizing* by creating a logical story or saying what they think the audience wants to hear, instead of the truth. These problems are discussed in more detail below.

Remembering. Memory fades over time, or, more accurately, it becomes more difficult to retrieve memories when cues related to those memories are no longer present and a succession of other events has captured one's attention and been mixed into memory. Some of this forgetting can be quite startling, such as the phenomenon of "highway hypnosis" when people suddenly realize they have been driving some distance, executing a complex routine, without any recollection of what they were doing (Natsoulas, 1970; see Ericsson & Simon, 1984).

Self-reports about decision processes are no different. Nisbett and Wilson (1977) offer a scathing critique of self-report techniques by demonstrating that the attributes of alternatives actually affecting decisions showed poor agreement with the attributes reported by subjects. For example, they asked customers in stores to evaluate articles of clothing, such as nylon stockings. The shoppers gave judgments of which was the highest quality and why they had made their decisions. There was a strong position effect—shoppers tended to pick the rightmost stocking, although all stockings were randomly arrayed—yet no one ever reported position as a factor in their judgments, and they denied the effect of position when asked directly. Nisbett and Wilson suggest that shoppers may have a habitual rule of moving from left to right and holding off on choice, but they are unaware of it. They summarize their review by stating:

> People often cannot report accurately on the effects of particular stimuli on higher order, inference-based responses. Indeed, sometimes they cannot report on the existence of critical stimuli, sometimes cannot report on the existence of their responses, and sometimes cannot even report that an inferential process of any kind has occurred. (p. 233)

Table 3.1 gives another illustration of the apparent difficulty people have in reporting about their decision processes. Although the broad interpretation of Nisbett and Wilson's results have been questioned frequently (Smith & Miller, 1978; Ericsson & Simon, 1984, pp. 25-30), the fact remains that subjects often cannot recall accurately or are unwilling to exert the effort necessary to recall.

Reconstructing. If people cannot recall all the details of an event, they may accurately report that "I just can't remember." It is very likely, however, that they will instead reconstruct their memories from the fragments and images they remember and their general knowledge. For example, a telephone survey asked how many times respondents had eaten in a restaurant in the last two months. In answering, only one quarter of the respondents tried to recall and count specific instances. The rest used some kind of inference strategy, such as estimating that they ate out about twice a week and multiplying by eight weeks to get an answer of sixteen (Burton & Blair, 1986). This may create a very plausible account, and may be convincing to both the questioner and the respondent; but it may or may not be accurate.

Decades of research on human memory reveal that reconstructions are based on information immediately present. For example, Loftus (1975; Loftus & Palmer, 1974) has shown that eyewitnesses to a traffic accident can be led to report different speeds when attorneys ask, "How fast was the car going when it *crashed* into the second car?" rather than "How fast was the car going when it *hit* the second car?" Fischhoff and Beyth (1975) showed that people incorrectly recalled their own past predictions about President Nixon's ground-breaking trip to the People's Republic of China as consistent with its actual success; their perfect "hindsight" was reconstructed as good "foresight."

Nisbett and Bellows (1977) demonstrated the same effect of reconstruction in experimental decision tasks. College students read an application portfolio of a woman applying for a counseling job and rated the

Table 3.1
Sample Interview Protocol

Nisbett and Schachter (1966) placed subjects in a laboratory experiment in which they were requested to take a series of electric shocks of steadily increasing intensity. They could refuse the shocks at any point in time. Subjects given a placebo pill and told the pill would produce heart palpitations, hand tremors, and other signs of fear took more shock than those not given a placebo. At the end of the study, each subject in the pill condition was interviewed or debriefed with questions designed to get at their decisions to take more shocks. The following series of questions and responses represent the debriefing questions and typical answers.

Q: "I notice that you took more shock than average. Why do you suppose you did?"

A: "Gee, I don't really know. . . . I used to build radios and stuff when I was 13 or 14, and maybe I got used to electric shock."

Q: "While you were taking the shock, did you think about the pill at all?"

A: "No, I was too worried about the shock."

Q: "Did it occur to you at all that the pill was causing some physical effects?"

A: "No, like I said, I was too busy worrying about the shock."

woman's intelligence, flexibility, sympathy, and how much they liked her. Students' self-reports of their priorities for these judgments coincided with predictions by other students of how the decisions would be made. Analyses of the decisions, however, showed that the self-reports were virtually useless for predicting the actual judgments of liking, flexibility, and sympathy. The only convergence was for judgments of intelligence, apparently because our culture provides us with a clear theory of the antecedents of intelligence. Thus, these decision makers (and the observers) were reconstructing judgments, not reporting actual decision processes.

Rationalizing. It should come as no great revelation that people do not always tell the truth. In one careful study of the accuracy of survey responses, 17% of respondents misreported their age, 25% were wrong about having registered and voted in the last election, and 40% were mistaken about whether or not they had contributed to the United Fund (Parry & Crossley, 1950). Part of this is a recall problem rather than deliberate misrepresentation. Those items with the most disagreement, however, are also those for which people are motivated to present a favorable impression of themselves to the interviewer. People tend to say they voted and contributed to charity when actually they did not; they rarely make the opposite error.

In an interesting series of studies, Ebbesen and Konecni (1982) compared several ways of asking judges how they set bail for defendants. One method was simply to ask them, which yielded answers referring to strength of community ties as the single most important factor. This result was consistent with their behavior in setting bail on hypothetical cases, and consistent with the recommendations of the pioneering Vera Institute of Justice on how judges should set bail. Analyses of the records of actual cases, however, showed a very different result: Judges based their bail decisions on the recommendations of the attorneys, and particularly on the recommendations of the prosecuting attorney. Community ties had only an indirect effect by influencing somewhat the recommendations of the attorneys. Judges know they do this, but they are unwilling to admit that they often take the lazy way out of evaluating cases, or that the real rule might be to maintain good working relationships with the attorneys.

Obtaining Accurate Self-Reports

In the process of making decisions, a rapid series of events occurs in our heads. Although we may have access to our foci of attention, sensations, emotions, evaluations, plans, and intermediate results of mental operations at the instant they are in consciousness, the rapid succession of thoughts makes it difficult to store all this in long-term memory. Furthermore, whatever is stored in long-term memory becomes more difficult to retrieve over time as subsequent experiences replace cues to that information and new, easily confused information is also mixed into memory. The way self-reports are elicited may encourage people to theorize rather than recall because recall is difficult (especially with the passage of time and a larger volume of intervening thoughts) or impossible (when people are asked about things they could not themselves recall, such as the difference between their own and others' behavior).

Ericsson and Simon (1984) suggest that "the accuracy of verbal reports depends on the procedures used to elicit them and the relation between the requested information and the actual sequence of heeded information" (p. 27). There are many kinds of self-report procedures differing in their effectiveness under various circumstances. For self-reports to be valid recollections, it makes sense for them to be as close in time as possible to the recollected material; for the procedure eliciting recall to be similar to the original situation; for the original event to have established a strong memory by being important, attracting conscious attention, or being repeated (Ericsson & Simon, 1984); and for the questions to be asked in an order that facilitates correct recall (Bradburn, Rips, & Shevell, 1987). Self-reports may also be valid reconstructions or theories when the influential factors are plausible, included in a priori theories, and there are no plausible noninfluential factors—that is, when the available theory happens to be correct (Nisbett & Wilson, 1977).

The quality of self-reports depends on the interviewer, the questions, and the situation, just as in any interview or questionnaire (Sudman & Bradburn, 1982). It should be emphasized that respondents must be motivated to be truthful, not simply helpful. In addition, the situation must be constructed so as to aid recall by avoiding distractions and proceeding in a logical order (e.g., a temporal order) that helps to access memory. Further, the researcher must avoid suggesting answers or otherwise providing a basis for an inaccurate reconstruction.

When to Use Informal Self-Reports

Informal self-reports are almost as easy to get as having a conversation. Their low cost makes them highly desirable investigative tools. There is virtually no technical skill necessary to use the method, although skilled interviewers and persons trained to probe and use multiple sources of information should produce higher quality results. It is not surprising, therefore, that the method is ubiquitous.

It is difficult to envision a research project that did not start by using the self-report method. We scout a prospective project by informally gathering opinions, identifying issues, learning the "ropes," and otherwise doing what we can to explore the situation. This is often the method of choice for exploratory research, for checking understanding, for generating hypotheses, and for enhancing the sophistication of research (Kidder & Judd, 1986). In this capacity, informal self-reports will continue to be used and are recommended highly.

The same logic posits the following question: Can we leave out self-reports from any study of decision making? It is easy to interpret Ebbesen and Konecni (1982) and Nisbett and Wilson (1977) as advocates for the use of "hard" data, and the avoidance of "soft" self-reports that can be misleading and biased. We would argue instead that self-reports are very valuable, even when they disagree with the results of other methods. It seems both scientifically sensible and fair to give those closest to problems a chance to give their interpretations, which should then be treated as skeptically as researchers treat their own hypotheses. Such data help to frame the issues early in research, ensure that one has not missed something important, provide one more test of understanding, and pose new questions about why self-reports sometimes differ from other sources of data.

Self-reports must be carefully designed and thought out, however, especially if they are to be the *only* source of information. In general, it seems wise to include other sources of information, such as records of past decisions, statements by other informants, behavior on controlled tasks, and so forth.

CASE STUDIES

Case studies are a collection of methods that approach each case as a unique and distinct entity, in what has been called an "idiographic approach" (Allport, 1937). The defining feature of case research is that the primary goal is to understand the case itself; only later might there be efforts to generalize from the case to broader principles. This is in contrast to the "nomothetic approach" that tries to discover and test general principles or laws that apply across cases, and may never learn or care much about an individual case. The case approach could draw on general principles, but they would be combined within the unique circumstances and context of each specific case.

Case studies tend to exhibit several common features: (1) considerable time is spent with each case; (2) the researcher attempts to understand the case in context, meaning that information about history and situation is collected; (3) verification checks directed at convergent validity are included by asking the same question in different ways, obtaining relevant information from other people or public records, and so forth; (4) the focus is on the internal consistency and meaningfulness of the information, not on a comparison to theories or expectations; and (5) the quality of the results depends on the ability of the researcher and the quality of the relationships established between researcher and respondents.

The nature of the "case" under consideration could be quite varied. The case could be a specific decision, such as Graham Allison's (1971) analysis of the Cuban missile crisis of 1962; a specific individual, as in the autobiographical book Richard Nixon wrote on his six key decisions (Nixon, 1962); or a group or organization, as in Powell's (1985) study of two companies in the publishing business including the processes by which manuscripts are chosen for publication. There are many varieties of case method, arising from journalism, ethnography, clinical psychology, historical analysis, the insights and experiences of consultants, and the collected experience of a society filled with "intuitive case analysts."

The goal of understanding cases in their richness demands a broad and flexible set of methods. Most typically, these methods are qualitative and range from informal to somewhat more formal. Case research often utilizes interviews with key actors and other informants, on-site observation of events, the collection of written documents, library research reading personal papers, biographers' reports, and whatever else clever researchers can think of as sources of information. Because there are usually only one or a handful of cases in a research study, statistical analyses rarely are helpful for summarizing the cases or drawing generalizations. Case analysis, however, may involve highly quantitative methods—for example, summarizing the kinds of decisions made by a single decision maker, or analyzing the financial situation of a company in order to understand its strategic choices.

Choosing Cases

The quality of case research depends primarily on the choice of cases and the perceptiveness and thoughtfulness of the case researcher. If little is known about the issues and potential cases, then a case may be chosen because it appears typical and thus is informative about most cases, or what Yin (1989) calls "revelatory." When past research provides some general understanding of cases, the case researcher may select a case that is unusual or extreme and therefore is intended to provoke some new thoughts.

It is advantageous to plan case research with comparisons in mind, for example, to research that has previously been done or to hypotheses drawn from well-formulated theories, or by selecting two or more cases that span some dimension of interest such as large versus small, expert versus novice, or successful versus unsuccessful. Comparisons provide what Yin (1989) calls *analytical generalization*: Cases may be revealed as similar to each other (literal replication), or different for predictable reasons that help develop theory (theoretical replication).

Of course, the choice of cases depends critically upon *access*. The feasibility of a case depends upon cooperation and logistics. The researcher's networks of friends and associates may be critical for gaining entry and conducting the research.

Discovery

Because case research is relatively unstructured, the approach is flexible enough to be adjusted to the peculiarities of individual cases, researchers, and research questions. To exploit this flexibility, the researcher must keep an open mind and remain alert to the unexpected. Often, the things that simply "turn up" may be more informative than the planned routines of data collection. For this reason, case researchers try to collect everything; they take copious notes and expand them immediately—a researcher's memory is no better than anyone else's!

On the other hand, the researcher risks getting swamped in details if the orienting questions and issues of the research are forgotten easily. It is essential to keep a careful record of one's own hypotheses, predictions, assumptions, and interpretations, as well as records of the data, in order to maintain some control over the research process and to pay attention to what does *not* fit in (see Campbell, 1979, for suggested "box scores"). Thus, good case researchers use their training and experience not only to develop specific techniques, but also to develop good research taste—a sense for what is important—that combines sensitivity, intuition, and good judgment.

An Example

Let us take as an example of case analysis Janis's (1982) study of several presidential policy decisions including five major fiascoes made by five different American presidents assisted by policy-making groups. In each instance, the members of the advisory group made "incredibly gross miscalculations about both the practical and moral consequences of their decisions" (p. viii) which, Janis argues, arose from a phenomenon called "groupthink." For comparison, Janis included two other decisions made by similar groups that exhibited good group process and realistic assessments of consequences.

Each case analysis looked in depth at the events and at the thought processes of the presidential advisors as they grappled with these decisions. The sources of information about these events and thoughts were, as Janis (1982) states,

> the contemporary and retrospective accounts by the group members themselves—minutes of the meetings, diaries, memoirs, letters, and prepared statements given to investigating committees—many of which are likely to have been written with an eye to the author's own place in history. (p. ix)

Janis focused on comparing decisions characterized by defective decision processes to those with good processes, and on identifying the causes, symptoms, and effects of groupthink. Thus, for example, learning that Robert Kennedy discouraged James Schlesinger from voicing doubts about the Bay of Pigs invasion plans ("Now is the time for everyone to get behind the President"), Janis labels this an instance of a "self-appointed mindguard." The net result is both a series of case studies—each a self-contained historical story—and a list of concepts that form a theory of the causes, effects, and cures associated with groupthink.

As a result of his selection and analysis of the cases, however, Janis's approach could be criticized for being overly confirmatory. He was searching for bad causes of bad outcomes, and good causes of good outcomes, that fit his notions. It seems clear that these seven decisions were not a random sample of all group policy decisions, but instead were selected to make a point from among decisions for which appropriate sources of information existed, yet which had the capability to enrich and deepen Janis's ideas about group decision making. He was not primarily interested in explaining how a particular unique decision was made in its entirety, nor in finding examples that contradicted the groupthink concept. Given a large body of evidence that suggests that people often look for confirmatory evidence and disregard inconsistent information (Nisbett & Ross, 1980), this fear seems realistic.

Varieties of Case Research

Case research—or any method, for that matter—can focus on various units of analysis, goals, and decision stages. As we discussed in Chapter 2, the unit of analysis could be a decision, a decision maker (whether group or individual), or a decision process such as prediction or information-seeking strategies. Yin (1989) provides a useful discussion of units of analysis in case research. The goal could be any combination of understanding, predicting, or controlling decision behavior. And, as we have seen, research could be oriented around a particular case, or around principles that are generalized across cases.

An example of case research based on studying individual decision makers is Isenberg's (1987) observations of 12 general managers of divisions within six multidivisional corporations. His objective was to find out how they make decisions, which we could label understanding or theory building because he sought to understand each decision maker, and to generalize across them to increase our understanding of principles of decision making. His methods included interviews and on-site observations of each general manager during several work days. At intervals during the work days, Isenberg intruded into the workflow by asking what the executive was doing and thinking about at that moment (a form of verbal protocol—see Chapter 5). His results and interpretation focus in part on the *interconnectedness* of decisions, how executives are looking at a field of problems and decisions and seeking to take actions that move several problems along simultaneously. Such results are most likely to emerge from a method that looks at the whole person in context.

In contrast, applied researchers are concerned more directly with the cases themselves because they are trying to solve here-and-now problems (the goal of control), or to teach the ways of solving real problems. Consultants, clinicians, and educators often have this type of case orientation. Sigmund Freud used this approach in trying to unlock the secrets of his clients and to effect cures. Journalists unravel the story of events in this manner (Levine, 1980); the Rogers Commission studied the *Challenger* disaster in this way; and biographers and historians have the same singular focus of attention. In the business world, the Harvard Business School uses the case method to train the reasoning skills of its students: Cases are analyzed and discussed, but the goal is to seek understanding and to be open to possibilities. There is no "right answer" or final assessment of the case, but some answers are acknowledged as being better than others.

Problems With Case Methods

The case literature is filled with accounts that may be little more than good stories or window dressing for the opinions of researchers. Sometimes, this is because the case researcher has accepted the "party line" given by one or more informants, and has failed to check deeply enough to verify this information. Researchers may even "go native," becoming well-socialized members of the case community and losing their research perspective. Or, more simply, they may pay too much attention to aspects of the rich and varied case material that support their own preconceived ideas, without considering systematically the implications of all the data—specifically, what does *not* fit in (Campbell, 1979).

The normal checks and balances of empirical research are greatly weakened in case research. Most cases are chosen by accident: the researcher happens to have a contact at the site, access was relatively easy to obtain, or for unknown reasons. The quality of the results depends on the abilities and diligence of the case researcher. No one is there to check whether the researcher has recorded field notes accurately, tried various interpretations, or talked to the right people in the right way. The ability to obtain sensitive "insider" information depends on the quality of the relationship between researcher and respondents; other researchers cannot evaluate this effectively. Furthermore, there is no demand for replication: Case researchers almost never redo a case someone else has examined, because novelty is one of the major contributions of case description, and consistency is not an absolute requirement for case research. Disagreements between case researchers who have studied the same case, if they arise at all, are typically explained as real change (therefore, two different cases) or as two different descriptions of the case, both of which are true.

The lesson for the budding case researcher is that a great deal of information can flow from the study of cases, and the case researcher must manage that process if the information is to be valid and useful. This means being explicit about what is being done, and why; being diligent about following good procedures such as keeping regular field notes; being forthright about preconceptions and hypotheses so that confirming and disconfirming information is noted carefully; and being disciplined about remaining faithful to the research questions without being so rigid that exciting opportunities are ignored.

SELF-REPORT AND CASE METHODS: A CONSUMER'S GUIDE

Our discussion of these two methods has suggested both advantages and disadvantages for each. We will elaborate on these by using the six criteria for evaluating methods that were proposed in Chapter 1: discovery, understanding, prediction, prescriptive control, confound control, and ease of use.

Self-Report

We have suggested that research projects frequently begin with questions addressed to decision makers or those who have some knowledge about how the decisions are made. This occurs because researchers need to orient themselves to new topics, to uncover issues and interesting phenomena, and to develop hypotheses about the principles that underlie decisions. We can therefore evaluate the self-report method as strong on the criterion of discovery, because it reveals possibilities and suggests ideas. It can be strong on understanding, because people can offer their underlying reasoning and opinions about the mechanisms and causes of the decisions. Such reports, however, may not be accurate. Finally, it is moderately strong on ease of use, except that the most difficult aspect is gaining access to the right respondents (see Chapter 7 for more on such practical issues).

The information obtained from self-reports, however, has to be carefully assessed. We would evaluate this method as somewhat low in confound control, because it is difficult to overcome or even assess the quality of responses without additional sources of information. As a result, it is also somewhat low in prediction and prescriptive control. With a great deal of care and technical expertise in the design of questions and the selection of respondents (toward more formal survey designs), it is possible to improve performance on these criteria, with the trade-off of making the technique more difficult and expensive.

Case Methods

For those interested in the richness of actual cases, in understanding a good story, staying close to naturalistic events, exploring new areas and discovering new phenomena, and applying our understanding to therapeutic ends, case research is an appropriate choice. Case methods therefore share with self-reports strength on the criteria of discovery and understanding. Because case methods usually incorporate a variety of data sources, they are potentially even stronger on these criteria.

Case methods are also strong on prediction and prescription for the cases that were studied. This is why case methods are so popular for therapeutic purposes. This strength is local, however, in the sense that generalization to other instances is problematic. Case methods are much weaker at creating generalizations than at understanding specific instances.

As Campbell (1979) has pointed out, case research does not have to be atheoretical—cases can disconfirm treasured hypotheses. Even so, their use in hypothesis testing remains rather clumsy, because researchers rarely keep explicit lists of their hypotheses (which may change as cases progress) and the relationship between these hypotheses and data observed. We express this as somewhat of a weakness in confound control.

Case research does make great demands on the researcher in terms of time, interpersonal skill, sensitivity, and vulnerability to the whims of those who control the case "turf." Although it may appear to be easy to do case research, it is far more difficult (and more infrequent) to do *good* case research. Yin (1989) asserts that "the demands of a case study on a person's intellect, ego, and emotions are far greater than those of any other research strategy" (p. 62). Thus, we would have to evaluate the case method as fairly difficult to employ well.

As we turn our attention to other research methods in the following chapters, we will identify methods in Chapters 4 and 5 that are appropriate for studying actual decisions and practicing decision makers, combining both relevance and rigor. In Chapter 6, we will see that researchers who use their own special materials and conduct research on their own turf (such as the laboratory) have much easier research management tasks. Such controlled methods are designed appropriately for addressing specific, well-structured research questions.

SKILL BUILDING

1. Suppose you have just been given a speeding ticket. In conversation with a friend, the friend reveals that he was also stopped for speeding recently, but was able to "talk his way out of it." You decide that you would like to know how the police decide whether or not to issue tickets.

   (a) How would you define your research interests, in terms of units, goal, and stages?

   (b) From whom would you like to get information? How would you get access to them? Why should they talk to you?

   (c) What questions would you like to ask?

   (d) How could you assess the quality of the responses?

   (e) Are there any other sources of data that you could obtain?

   (f) What sort of generalizations or conclusions would you hope to state at the end of your research? What form would your "answers" take: quantitative models, qualitative descriptions, lists of factors, or what?

2. Let's suppose that you work for an organization that has recently adopted new computer workstations for electronic mail, word processing, and so forth. How could you find out how this adoption decision was made? Think of this decision as a case.

   (a) To whom could you talk? Who would know something meaningful about the decision? (Hint: Not just people inside the organization!)

(b) What other sources of information might be useful?

(c) What role might be played by theories in suggesting categories of data, kinds of interpretations, and ways to organize the research?

(d) Who would be interested in knowing about the adoption decision? Of what use would the resulting description be, and to whom?

4

Weighted-Additive Models

INTRODUCTION

Remember our stockbroker from the last chapter? Imagine that we notice that she has been a doing a lot of trading in our portfolio, selling many of our shares after holding them for a very brief period of time, and buying different stocks. Furthermore, it seems that all this activity is producing very unfavorable returns. Although she claims that her decisions are based on sound principles, we wonder whether she might be unduly influenced by her short-term income from brokerage commissions. We would like to know how she makes her trading decisions without relying on her stated reasoning, because she may be "selling" instead of reporting, or she may be unable to give an accurate report of her judgments.

In this chapter, we present a set of techniques that build a formal representation or *weighted-additive model* of the decision maker's behavior. In theory, such models can capture the decision maker's preferences. To the extent we are successful, a weighted-additive model can stand in for the decision maker, predicting what decisions would be made and offering explanations in terms of values or preferences.

Weighted-additive models are sometimes referred to as input-output models because they represent the basic structure of a decision program as the relationship between inputs (a set of alternatives described by attributes) and output (evaluations of alternatives made by the decision maker). For example, each stock has a price-earnings ratio, level of volatility, and so forth. Weighted-additive models relate this attribute information about each stock to the decision maker's choices or willingness to buy. These overall evaluations, which we will call Y_i (the subscript i refers to the alternative), are expressed as a rule or mathematical function (f) of the attributes which we will call X_{ij} (the subscript j indicates that there are many attributes). Thus, all these models share a common abstract form:

$$Y_i = f(X_{ij}). \qquad [4.1]$$

Because f is usually expressed as a set of weights applied to the attributes—and a summation of the weighted attributes—we have called these models *weighted-additive models*. When required, these evaluations can be converted into choices by assuming that decision makers pick the alternative with the highest Y_i.

The goal of these techniques is to identify f by analyzing attributes and decisions, but without looking directly at any of the intervening steps in the decision process. In Chapter 5, we will examine methods that gather more direct observations of mental processes, and in Chapter 6 we look at methods that use highly controlled inputs in order to infer decision processes.

TYPES OF WEIGHTED-ADDITIVE MODELS: AN ORGANIZATIONAL SCHEME

Many different kinds of weighted-additive models exist, differing in their origins, assumptions, goals, and techniques. Individual members of this "family" of models were developed and used in diverse disciplines such as psychology, operations research, marketing, and engineering. These disciplines use different terminologies, creating a Tower of Babel in which real relationships among methods are difficult to discern. Further, some methods set as their goal to help people make better decisions, while other methods try to predict a decision maker's choices and remain largely silent about their quality. There often is debate about which model is better, and advocates can adhere to their beliefs with almost religious fervor.

To overcome this confusion, we will introduce different models by providing a common language and framework. We cannot settle historical arguments, nor provide exhaustive lists of the similarities among weighted-additive models. Instead, we can organize our descriptions so that you can judge which is most useful for your own applications. In this sense, we are attempting to supply a kind of consumer's guide to different modeling techniques, helping to identify techniques that are appropriate for given situations.

Alternative-Focused Versus Attribute-Focused Techniques

A major theoretical and practical issue in decision making is whether preferences are best thought of as properties of alternatives or of attri-

Table 4.1
Alternative-Focused and Attribute-Focused Approaches

	Approach	
	Alternative-Focused	*Attribute-Focused*
Attribute Values	Assumed	Elicited
Attribute Weights	Calculated	Elicited
Combination Rule	Assumed or limited variety tested	Assumed
Preferences for Alternatives	Elicited	Calculated

butes. Can we best understand decisions by studying reactions to alternatives (cars, for example), or reactions to the attributes from which they are built (e.g., styling, acceleration)? In other words, does Jim want to purchase the Corvette in the showroom, or a powerful red sports car with the model name Corvette?

Our first theme partitions different methods by what they require as input from the decision maker. *Alternative-focused* techniques use, as input, judgments of the alternatives—the Y_i in Equation 4.1. From these stated judgments (or from choices among alternatives), the researcher can infer the contributions of the component attributes. In contrast, *attribute-focused* techniques ask decision makers questions about each of the attributes—the X_{ij} in [4.1]. For example, we can ask car purchasers about the importance of fuel economy, or financial analysts about the importance of risk. Then, overall preferences for alternatives are calculated from the values placed on the separate attributes for each alternative, combined according to an assumed decision rule.[1] The distinctions between alternative-focused and attribute-focused models are summarized in Table 4.1.

Descriptive Versus Prescriptive Models

Our second organizing theme examines *why* the analyst is studying the decision. The goal of *descriptive* models is to understand and to predict choices. To do this they uncover decision makers' perceptions of the attributes, X_{ij}, and the nature of the function, f, that underlie preferences.

Descriptive models normally are successful if they: (1) explain existing judgments, and (2) provide adequate predictions of subsequent judgments. They do not strive to improve the quality of those decisions.

In contrast, *prescriptive* models have a different goal—helping decision makers to make better decisions. They change the decision process by clarifying perceptions of the attributes associated with alternatives, X_{ij}, and by altering the decision rule, f, to avoid inconsistencies, confusions, or biases on the part of decision makers.

Real Versus Hypothetical Decisions

The third organizing theme is whether the research investigates real decisions, including actual decision makers, and authentic materials and information—or, to achieve greater experimental control—uses hypothetical decisions (which may appear realistic) constructed by the researchers to serve specific purposes. Realism is enhanced by ecological designs that select representative decisions with typical relationships among variables (Brunswik, 1955), by richly detailed decision situations, and by real consequences attached to decision outcomes.

One of the virtues of weighted-additive models is that they can be applied to either real or hypothetical decisions. For example, these methods can be used with actual decisions such as stock recommendations or personnel hiring. The same techniques can also be used to examine more or less realistic situations, such as real decision makers with authentic materials, but no real consequences; or role-playing students with excerpted or hypothetical materials; or any other combination.

Although it may appear that "mundane realism" or "face validity" is essential to the study of decision making, the key issue is the attitude of the decision maker: Is the decision maker adequately involved, properly informed, and able to act in ways that relate to the reason why these decisions are being studied? This kind of "experimental realism" (Carlsmith, Ellsworth, & Aronson, 1978) or "subjective realism" obviously is present in actual decision making. The use of hypothetical stimuli does not necessarily create unrealistic preferences; abbreviated or hypothetical situations can be very "real" to their participants. At times, hypothetical decisions are preferable because they can give clearer answers to some questions, and they make it possible to study unique, rare, or future decisions that have no available data bases for study.

The sections that follow will be organized around the first two themes of attribute versus alternative focus and descriptive versus prescriptive goals. Throughout the chapter, we will focus on research that uses actual decisions or highly realistic approximations of real decisions. Research using highly controlled and typically less realistic materials and designs will be discussed in Chapter 6. We will first discuss methods that have an alternative focus, and then methods that have an attribute focus. Within each type we will discuss models that have descriptive and prescriptive uses. For each combination, we will present a prototypical model and discuss it in some depth, including an example of its application and an overview of related methods. We will end the chapter with a summary of the advantages and disadvantages of each method.

ALTERNATIVE-FOCUSED METHODS

Alternative-focused methods use observations of a decision maker's past choices and judgments to infer what drove the decision. By comparing how alternatives differ on the known attributes, and how these differences affect choices, these methods build a model of the decision maker. An advantage of these methods is that they do not require either the decision maker's self-insight or cooperation. In fact, they can be used without the decision maker's awareness. All that is needed is: (1) knowledge of the actual alternatives and attributes available to the decision maker; (2) observations of the decision maker's preferences in this set of alternatives; and (3) statistical model-building techniques.

Descriptive Models with an Alternative Focus:
Linear Models of Judgment

Although there are many ways to relate the characteristics of alternatives to observed preferences, the most common techniques employ a weighted linear combination of attributes. Continuing to formalize our notation, we use Y_i to stand for the subjective judgments made by the decision maker, such as whether a given player should be selected to play in the All-Star game in the National Basketball Association. For example, Y_1 could be the judged All-Star quality of the first basketball player, Y_2 the quality of the second, and so forth. We label the attributes associated with the players X_{ij} : X_{11} would be the points per game for the first player, X_{12} would be the number of assists for the first player, and so forth.

Once we know the set of alternatives (basketball players), the attributes that matter, and the values for each player on each attribute, what we have to find is the decision rule, f. Typically, researchers start with a *linear model* that adds up the values on the attributes (the X_{ij}'s), weighting each of them to give the best prediction of preference for the Y_i's. This can be represented by the following equation:

$$Y_i = b_0 + (b_1 \times X_{i1}) + (b_2 \times X_{i2}) + \ldots + (b_n \times X_{in}). \quad [4.2]$$

This equation is saying, in essence: "To predict Y_i (the rating of Player i as an NBA All-Star), simply take so much (b_1) of X_{i1} (their points per game), add so much (b_2) of X_{i2} (number of assists)," and so forth. The b coefficients capture both the units in which the X's are expressed and the relative importance of the X's. The b_0 is simply a starting point that helps account for the average quality of players.

Typically, decision researchers use regression as one way of establishing a mapping between attributes and preferences. Regression has many statistical advantages, including a complete set of statistics for evaluating a model of the decision maker and deciding if it is a good one. While a complete exposition of regression is beyond the scope of this book, the curious reader is referred to Neter, Wasserman, and Kuntner (1985).

Table 4.2 provides a more complete description of the steps involved in creating a regression model of decision making, in this case examining loan officers' judgments of credit worthiness on loan applications.

It may seem that linear models of decision making are a dumb idea. Our own judgments don't feel like mathematical combinations: we don't usually add up different attributes, but rather expect the impact of one variable to depend on the values of the others. For example, a sportswriter might think that the importance of shot-blocking and rebounds in selecting an All-Star would be very different for centers than for guards. In fact, both novices and experts report that their decision rules contain interactions—configural combinations of the input cues in which the impact of one depends on the value of another. We might also expect nonlinear relationships (log and power functions) between cues and decisions. Knowing this, we might guess that regression models are bound to be poor representations of decision makers' rules and that the assumption of linear relationships is wrong. This would seem even more true for complex decisions made by experts such as doctors or financial analysts.

Surprisingly, though, simple regression models using linear combinations of three to five attributes often predict decision makers' preferences very well and can be very useful. Seldom can we make significantly more accurate predictions by including configural combinations or terms in the model. Because they are relatively accurate predictors of choices, these

Table 4.2
Steps in Constructing Regression Models of Judgment with Example

Assume that you are modeling the decisions made by a loan officer who evaluates mortgage applications on a three-point scale: (1) do not issue a loan, (2) perhaps issue a loan, and (3) definitely issue a loan. To construct a policy-capturing or regression model, one should follow these steps:

1. *Carefully define the choice problem.* We should have a clear idea of what judgment we are modeling. In our example, we are assuming that we are modeling judgments of risk, rather than who will be a good customer for other reasons (e.g., they do a lot of other business with the bank).

2. *Identify which attributes are available to the decision maker.* We need to know what information the decision maker can consider, preferably coded in quantitative form. We can find out what information is available to the decision maker by asking representative decision makers or by examining the file folders from which decisions are made. In our example, the loan officer might know the applicants' ages, occupations, years living in the community, number of previous loans repaid, and number of times late with auto payments. If we wanted to include some non-numeric information in our model, we might ask the decision maker to rate it on a numeric scale. For example, our loan officer might rate applicants' future job security on a 7-point scale labeled from very uncertain to very certain. If there are attributes that are categorical, it is possible to represent them with "dummy" variables (see Neter, Wasserman, & Kuntner, 1985).

3. *Collect a set of preferences with typical alternatives.* We need to collect data about the decision maker's preferences using a typical or representative set of alternatives. In our example, we might simply observe which loan applications fall into each of the three categories during the course of several weeks, and note the values of the attributes for each application. The number of cases will typically be large, at least 10 for each variable we include in the model. Fifty to 100 cases would be a reasonable minimum.

4. *Other ways to collect preferences.* Instead of collecting preferences from a concurrent set of judgments, it is possible to get preferences from past decisions or hypothetical decisions. Records of past decisions could be used to gather a usable set of preferences. This has the advantage of being unobtrusive, but prevents the use of additional ratings by the decision maker (unless the decision maker goes back over the cases, which creates problems of retrospective judgment). Or, hypothetical cases could be constructed and rated, avoiding the problem of waiting for suitable decisions to happen, but reintroducing some of the problems of self-report. Chapter 6 provides a more detailed discussion of the use of hypothetical decisions.

5. *Construct a model.* We can then regress the variables that the loan officer can consider against the likelihood that a loan will be issued. In this case the outcomes (Y) will be coded from 1 (do not issue) to 3 (definitely issue). Ideally, we would want a continuous scale for Y. For ordinal data, ordinal regression is most appropriate. In cases with yes/no decisions, special statistical techniques such as logistic regression and discriminant analysis are needed to build the model.

(Continued)

Table 4.2 (Continued)

6. *Evaluate the model.* We get a first hint of the quality of the representation when we see how well the model predicts the outcomes it has been given. One measure, R^2, tells us the percent of variance in the judgments the model describes. To further assess the adequacy of the model, we may cross-validate by using this model to predict a new set of judgments. If the model did a suitable job of predicting the preferences of the loan officer, then we have developed a reasonable representation of the decision maker's preferences. As discussed, we might even want to replace the decision maker with this model!

7. *Elaborate or further test the model.* Simple linear models usually do a good job, but there are ways to check whether a better model is achievable. One strategy is to compose nonlinear terms (for example, is income, or a log-transform of income, or income and income × income, a better predictor) and configural terms (cross-products of two predictors to test for interactions) to see if these improve the model. A second strategy is to compute the residuals (actual decisions-predicted decisions) and correlate them with the actual decisions to see if there is systematic variance to explain (thus justifying adding nonlinear and configural terms). A third strategy is to confront decision makers with their models and solicit comments and suggestions, which could be tested by adding new predictors.

---

models are sometimes called *policy capturing* since they "capture" or represent the implicit policy or rules by which an individual or an organization makes decisions (Hammond, Stewart, Brehmer, & Steinmann, 1975).

An Example: Describing How Stock Prices Are Predicted

Wright (1979) was interested in how financial analysts use information for predicting stock prices. In his study, Stanford University MBA students in finance predicted the future percentage change in price of 50 actual stocks. The 50 companies were from one industry sector, with minimum sales of $20 million and careful attention paid to the representativeness of the stock data. The predictions were based on four actual attributes of each stock: percentage change in earnings, volatility of earnings over time, percentage of earnings distributed in cash, and a measure of risk based on capital asset pricing theory. Although Wright looks at several groups of judges, we will concentrate on one group of 12 students who had almost finished their MBA course work and were completing a course on contemporary stock market theory. The subjects knew they were making real predictions about real stocks, although company identities were withheld. To make this study more realistic, they were motivated by prizes up to $25 for the most accurate predictions.

Each stock analyst was presented with the four attributes of each stock, and asked to predict its price change. Wright built a unique linear regression model of each analyst:

$$\begin{aligned}
\text{Predicted price change} = b_0 \\
+ (b_1 \times \text{Change in earnings}) \\
+ (b_2 \times \text{Volatility of earnings}) \\
+ (b_3 \times \text{Percentage of earnings paid out}) \\
+ (b_4 \times \text{Risk}).
\end{aligned} \qquad [4.3]$$

Wright found that the models provided reasonably good accounts of these budding financiers' judgments. About one half of the variance in judgments was accounted for by the models. While this is not spectacularly high, it is typical of such modeling efforts.

Furthermore, the coefficients of the models tell us about the relationship between the predictor variables and the model. A positive coefficient tells us that an increase in this attribute causes an increase in predicted price, while a negative coefficient tells us that an increase in this attribute causes a decrease in predicted price. We must be especially careful in interpreting the size of the coefficients, because they depend on the measurement scale of each attribute, as well as their "importance." For example, risk is measured between −1 and +1, while the percentage of earnings paid goes from 0 to 100. To compare these we can look at standardized regression weights, which equalize the differences by multiplying the unstandardized weights by the standard deviation of the variable.

Let's look at what the prediction equation might have been for one of these decision makers, looking first at the raw (unstandardized) regression weights:[2]

$$\begin{aligned}
\text{Predicted price change} = (1.45 \times \text{Change in earnings}) \\
- (.003 \times \text{Volatility of earnings}) \\
- (.349 \times \text{Percentage of earnings paid out}) \\
+ (.08 \times \text{Risk}).
\end{aligned} \qquad [4.4]$$

The model says that for a particular stock that changed earnings by 10%, had earnings volatility of 20%, paid out 16% of earnings, and had a risk index of .50, the prediction can be made by following the formula

$(1.45 \times 10) - (.003 \times 20) - (.349 \times 16) + (.08 \times .50)$, giving a result of 8.9%. In the same manner, the model tells us how the stock analyst might react to new stocks that were not presented in the original set. By plugging in the values of a new stock for each of the variables in the equation above, we can generate a prediction for unseen stocks.

The advantage of standardizing the regression weights is that the relative importance of the attributes becomes more readily apparent. The above equation, with standardized weights, is:

$$\text{Predicted price change} = (.547 \times \text{Change in earnings})$$
$$- (.045 \times \text{Volatility of earnings})$$
$$- (.219 \times \text{Percent of earnings paid out})$$
$$+ (.001 \times \text{Risk}). \qquad [4.5]$$

Standardization translates all variables into a standard unit scale based on standard deviations. In this example, for every increase of one standard unit in the change in earnings, predictions of price increase by .547 standard units. Similarly, if a company pays out one standard deviation above the mean in earnings, this stock analyst would lower the predicted price by .219 standard units. Interpreting these standardized weights as a measure of the relative importance should be done with caution, because weights are still influenced by the distribution of data on the scales and their intercorrelations among predictors (when the attributes are correlated, the weights are increasingly ambiguous; in Wright's study, the four attributes had an average correlation of .413).

An interesting result from Wright's (1979) work relates directly to our original question about our stockbroker who was making trades that did not seem to correspond to her self-reported decision rule. Wright asked the decision makers what weights they placed on the four attributes, by having them allocate 100 points among the attributes. The weights they reported were quite different from those revealed by the models, although more knowledgeable subjects appeared to have more self-insight. As we will see in Chapter 5, decision makers' self-reports are not always as veridical as we might hope (e.g., Cook & Stewart, 1975; Nisbett & Wilson, 1977).

Trained financial analysts should use much more complicated decision rules than what is expressed in the linear regression model; the simple model may fail to capture an important part of judgment. We can test this by looking at the error in the model (the "residuals" in regression) and see what relationship, if any, it has with actual price changes. In Wright's study, the error in the linear model is not closely related to price changes: it accounts for less than 4% of the variance in price changes. In other words, there is not much more of the students' predictions that can be modeled. For this reason, making the model more complicated by adding combinations of variables—interaction terms—doesn't improve the model of the decision makers very much. Thus, the "dumb" linear model not only does a surprisingly good job of modeling these financial analysts, but whatever it misses does not seem to matter in predicting what they will say about future stock prices (in other words, the error is really "noise").

To summarize, Wright's results (which are typical of applications in business, medicine, psychology, public policy, and many other domains) showed that a simple linear model produced a relatively accurate prediction of decision makers' preferences, capturing almost all of the valid parts of the decision makers' judgments.

Alternative-Focused Models with Prescriptive Goals

We turn now to models that have a different goal: better decisions. Unlike descriptive models, prescriptive models don't necessarily describe the decision makers. Because decision makers are fallible, prescriptive models try to prevent them from making mistakes, such as getting confused when combining information about multiple attributes. We will consider the possibility that various kinds of "dumb" regression models might make better decisions than unaided decision makers.

In the example of Wright's study of stock price prediction (discussed above), the models of the student analysts made better predictions of the actual price changes in the 50 stocks than did the students themselves. Such models are called "bootstrapping models" because the decision makers' own judgments can be used to "pull the decision makers up by their own bootstraps" (Goldberg, 1968). This result has been replicated in many real-world tasks ranging from security analysis (Ebert & Kruse, 1978) to medical judgment (Einhorn, 1972).

The basic reason for this phenomenon is that the linear regression model is consistent in representing some of what the decision makers consider important. The model never gets confused, never makes wild guesses, never gets distracted by a novel piece of information, and never gets tired. Apparently, decision makers are inconsistent enough in following their own implicit rules that they do worse than their own models.

An Example: Improving the
Graduate Admissions Process

When the second author of this book applied to graduate schools in psychology, he was surprised by the application form supplied by one well-known school—the University of Colorado. Along with the normal material—extolling the virtues of the program, its faculty, and the attractions of living in Boulder, Colorado—came an interesting card which outlined a formula that the graduate school used for evaluating candidates. It asked prospective students to add up their grade point average, standardized test scores, and number of science courses taken, first multiplying each by a constant. The card then gave a rule to translate the total score into a figure representing the likelihood of admission. Above one total score the chances were very good, whereas below another cutoff level applicants had little hope. Intermediate scores meant admission was possible, but not certain.

This model was constructed using a statistical analysis of the way the faculty made admission decisions, based on hundreds of applicants they had evaluated over the past several years. The model related the attributes (e.g., grade point average) to preferences (admit versus reject) using an alternative-based linear model. It was alternative based because the decision makers gave their overall preferences for each alternative (applicants), and the weights for the attributes were determined by the regression analysis. Notice that the steps to build the model are quite similar for a descriptive or prescriptive model: What matters is how the model is used. Notice also that this is a model of a group decision, rather than of individual decision makers.

In this situation, the faculty had decided that their decision rule was so explicit that it could be shared with applicants. By making the rule public, the graduate program had decided that it could help applicants with their own decisions of whether or not to apply, and save itself the time of evaluating applicants who had very little chance of admission.

Dawes (1971) reports that a similar linear model could screen 55% of all applicants to the University of Oregon's doctoral program in psychology, without rejecting anyone who would have been admitted by the committee. Dawes' model to predict the admission committee's ratings (on a 5-point scale) of student desirability was:

$$\text{Rating} = -4.17 + (.0032 \times \text{GRE}) + (1.02 \times \text{GPA}) + (.0791 \times \text{QI}) \quad [4.6]$$

where GRE was total Graduate Record Examination score, GPA was the overall undergraduate grade point average, and QI was a crude six-point index of the quality of the candidate's undergraduate school, obtained from a standard reference.[3] Note that these are unstandardized weights, and that the different sizes of the coefficients reflect differences in both importance and scale of the three attributes. For example, .0032 weights GRE totals that range from 400 to 1700, while the 1.02 weights GPAs that vary between 0 and 4. To predict the rating (and subsequent success) of a new applicant with a GRE score of 1300, a GPA of 3.6, and a QI of 5 we would calculate the rating from the formula $-4.17 + (.0032 \times 1300) + (1.02 \times 3.6) + (.0791 \times 5)$ as 4.06, which would be a very respectable rating on the 5-point scale.

Related Techniques: Actuarial Models

If our concern is to build a model that will make a better decision, then we do not necessarily need to study actual decision makers. Given a set of outcomes or performance criteria, we can build a linear model that relates the attributes to the outcomes without an intervening predictive judgment. These models are often termed *environmental* or *actuarial* models because they model the relationships found in the real world. In our graduate admissions example, Dawes (1973) had records for students who had been admitted to the program, including their actual performance in the program. A regression model was built to predict actual performance from the attributes, and this linear combination of the same three attributes was a much stronger predictor of performance than were the judgments of the admissions committee. Interestingly, the admissions committee seemed to pay too much attention to GRE scores and too little attention to the quality of the undergraduate institution.

Such actuarial models are commonplace in business today. For example, if you have applied for credit, a linear model probably played an important role in deciding whether or not your application was approved. The model probably considered your occupation, income, debt obligations, credit history, and other legally permissible factors. If anyone you know has ever been audited by the IRS, they may have been selected by a model designed to predict where additional revenues might be found. While knowing that a model picked you for an audit won't make the experience any more pleasant, you might at least feel less personally persecuted.

Over and over again, linear models have been proven more accurate than human decision makers doing the same tasks. Whether we use actuarial models based on real world outcomes or bootstrapping models based on the judgments of decision makers, this surprising result has been verified in many domains (see the classic review by Dawes, 1979). Dawes, Faust, and Meehl (1989) report that in about 100 comparisons of actuarial linear models to human experts, the linear model was superior in all but a handful of the cases (the exceptions were mostly medical tasks in which well-developed theory outpredicts limited statistical expertise). Because the model is not always better, we do not recommend automatically replacing the human decision maker; we do recommend that you compare models to the judgments of your expert(s).

Description and Prescription:
The Lens Model

Ken Hammond and his colleagues (Hammond, Stewart, Brehmer, & Steinmann, 1975) have developed the "Lens Model," which combines descriptive models of the decision maker and the prescriptive models of the environment as an overall approach to the improvement of decision making performance. Wright's (1979) study of stock price predictions and Dawes's (1973) study of graduate admissions are excellent examples of the Lens Model: both descriptive models of decision makers and actuarial or prescriptive models of outcome criteria are developed and compared for content, quality, and consistency. The results are used to learn more about decision making, and to make better decisions.

A Note On Equal-Weight Models

Sometimes, we have to make decisions when there is no available information about actual outcomes (from which to make an actuarial model) and no prior judgments by decision makers (from which to make a bootstrapping model). An equal-weight model requires only a list of predictor attributes and the direction of their relationship to outcomes— obtained, perhaps, by asking some experts. Such models look just like actuarial models, except that the *standardized* coefficients are all *equal*. In other words, we standardize all of the attributes by dividing the different scales by their standard deviation.[4] If we did not do this, attributes with wide ranges would be overweighted.

Although such models seem incredibly simple-minded, they often do a surprisingly good job at a very low cost. In Dawes's (1971) study of graduate admissions, an equal-weight model did better than the admissions committee! Einhorn and Hogarth (1975) recommend that when the number of actual outcomes or decisions is small (fewer than 50 to 100 data points to analyze), an equal-weight model is preferred to either bootstrapping or actuarial models. Equal-weight models work because they usually are quite robust (that is, resistant) to errors in specifying weights (Dawes & Corrigan, 1974; von Winterfeldt & Edwards, 1986), and therefore frequently provide a reasonable approximation of the true weights.

ATTRIBUTE-FOCUSED METHODS

Attribute-focused approaches are a family of methods that predict preferences or overall evaluations based on decision makers' perceptions of the attributes possessed by alternatives. These methods elicit from the decision makers their perceptions of the alternatives on the attributes (X_{ij}) and the importance of the attributes (b_j) (see Table 4.1 and Equation 4.2). The separate judgments about the input attributes are combined using an a priori decision rule, usually a linear model, into overall preferences for each alternative (Y_i).

Descriptive Models with an Attribute Focus:
Attitude Models of Preference

One attribute-focused technique that is widely used in marketing is the simple form of the Fishbein model (Ajzen & Fishbein, 1975). This model predicts attitudes toward a behavior (e.g., buying a Toyota is good or bad) by eliciting a set of beliefs about the likely consequences of the behavior (e.g., if I buy a Toyota, I will be getting a car with high gas mileage), each of which can be evaluated positively or negatively (i.e., high gas mileage is desirable). Although developed as a model of attitudes, it has been used extensively in marketing as a model to predict choices (see Wilkie & Pessimier, 1973).

The decision rule is:

$$A_i = (B_{i1} \times a_1) + (B_{i2} \times a_2) + \ldots + (B_{in} \times a_n) \qquad [4.7]$$

where A_i is the attitude toward an alternative (such as a Toyota), B_{ij} is the strength of the belief that choosing alternative i will lead to a particular consequence (such as good gas mileage), and a_j is the evaluation of the consequence (how desirable is good gas mileage?)

To understand the Fishbein model as an attribute-based model, we must recognize that the "attributes" in this case are the expected consequences of selecting an alternative. In practice, the original terms used by Fishbein often take on the interpretation that B_{ij} is a belief about the position of the alternative on an attribute (something like a value), and a_j the experience (or weight) attached to that belief (see Wilkie & Pessimier, 1973, for a discussion).

An Example: Preference for Soft Drinks

If we were trying to predict preferences for soft drinks such as Coke, Pepsi, and 7-Up, we would try to predict attitudes toward these drinks, which would be labeled A_1 (Coke), A_2 (Pepsi), and so forth. To predict attitudes, we need to identify the important attributes, which usually is done by looking at past research and asking people to list the things they like or dislike about soft drinks (in this case). Then the most frequently mentioned attributes (usually about seven) are retained for further study. For example, B_{11} might be the perceived thirst-quenching ability of Coke, and a_1 the importance associated with thirst-quenching.

Measurement of both importance weights and attribute positions is often done on seven-point bipolar scales. For the soft-drink example these might look like:

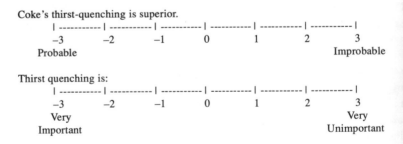

Coke's thirst-quenching is superior.

| ----------- | ----------- | ----------- | ----------- | ----------- | ----------- |
-3 -2 -1 0 1 2 3
Probable   Improbable

Thirst quenching is:

| ----------- | ----------- | ----------- | ----------- | ----------- | ----------- |
-3 -2 -1 0 1 2 3
Very   Very
Important   Unimportant

Once the attribute positions and weights are measured, the attitude toward each soft drink would be computed by multiplying each attribute position by the corresponding weight, and adding up the resultant cross-products. Purchase rates are assumed to be a direct result of attitude toward the product: given a choice among soft drinks, a shopper should choose whichever brand has the most positive attitude.

Although the Fishbein model has been historically important, it has faded in popularity among decision researchers because of several criticisms associated with its application. First, multiplying the beliefs by their strengths can be troublesome because people use scales like these in different ways: Some people use the middle range, while others respond to everything (including questionnaires) with extremes. It is hard to separate differences in response style from true differences in beliefs about the attributes. Researchers sometimes adjust responses to eliminate scale effects by standardizing each subject's responses: subtracting the mean and dividing by the standard deviation of each scale. Even so, it is problematic to compare the importance of beliefs for different groups of people, or make predictions for aggregates of people. A second problem concerns halo effects: For well-known brands, it is not clear if the overall attitudes (A_i) arise from the beliefs (B_{ij}) or rather that the overall attitudes create the beliefs. Finally, while first suggested as an attitude model, the model has been applied far beyond its original bounds; for example, to predict consumer choice. While the model has done surprisingly well (Sheppard, Harwick, & Warshaw, 1988), its usefulness as a decision theory is correspondingly weakened.

Prescriptive Models With Attribute Focus: Decision Analysis

Decision analysis is based on the assumption that decision makers want to follow good decision rules, but are unable to because of lack of knowledge, or "cognitive overload" in the face of complex situations. These decision rules are based on economic theories such as subjective expected utility theory (von Neumann & Morgenstern, 1953) and mathematical principles such as Bayes' Theorem (Edwards, 1961).

While psychologists have spent much effort attacking expected utility as an overly rational description of actual decision making, decision analysts interpret the attacks on the descriptive adequacy of the theory as a criticism of people for failing to "follow" the theory! Decision analysts take the prescriptive theory and human failings as evidence of a need for decision engineering.

To address these human failings, decision analysts use a "divide and conquer" strategy: The decision maker answers a series of simpler questions about the attributes that compose real or hypothetical alternatives, and their priorities or weights. The decision analyst constructs a representation of the decision maker's preferences, based on an a priori decision rule drawn from normative theory and therefore more accurate (in theory) than the decision maker's own rule. This representation is then used to aid the decision maker in actual complex decision situations to make better decisions.

Decision analysis tends to use more sophisticated methods than the Fishbein model discussed above. In multiple attribute utility theory (MAUT) (von Winterfeldt & Edwards, 1986), for example, a more careful consideration of weighting questions is achieved through the successive ratio method. The decision maker first rank orders the attributes in terms of importance. Notice that this forces the decision maker to look carefully at comparisons of attributes, something not done by the Fishbein model. After the rank ordering, the decision maker is asked how much more important the first attribute is than the second, with the response typically given as a ratio. By repeating this process across attributes, a complete set of attribute weights is gathered. These weights are typically scaled so that they sum to 1.

The techniques that we have discussed so far have assumed linear effects of each attribute. For example, we assumed that an increase of 1% in rate of return for a stock will have the same impact on the evaluation of that stock, whether that increase raises the overall return from 0% to 1%, or from 56% to 57%. There clearly are situations like this where important nonlinearities exist, so that the increases are more important for small values than for large.

MAUT and its cousins produce a scaling of the X_i to account for these nonlinearities. Compare the form of the linear regression models that we have used previously to this new form:

$$Y_i = b_0 + b_1 \times u(x_{i1}) + b_2 \times u(x_{i2}) + \ldots + b_n \times u(x_{in}). \quad [4.8]$$

Here again, the overall evaluation is constructed by the weight multiplied by the value, but the value is now a function of the actual X_i's termed a utility function. Constructing this function requires cooperation and careful thought on the part of the decision maker.

The techniques used for constructing utilities are beyond the scope of this book, but the interested reader should look at Keeney and Raiffa (1976) and von Winterfeldt and Edwards (1986). These references also present techniques for incorporating uncertainty in the values of attributes, and provide numerous examples of business and public policy applications of decision analysis. Extremely complex decisions have been analyzed, such as the thirty-year plan for airport development in Mexico City.

Example: Evaluating New Computer Systems.

Grochow (1972, 1973) interviewed systems programmers about their usage patterns and objectives for general time-sharing systems. They reported four attributes as most important: (1) response time to simple requests such as editing and directory listings; (2) response time to computation-bound requests such as compiling programs; (3) percentage of the time that the system was available for logging in; and (4) reliability. Notice that these attributes refer to user satisfaction; choosing among systems would also involve cost calculations.

The researcher then assessed utility functions over the first three attributes, assuming that reliability had to be sufficiently high. The three attributes were measured by average number of seconds to satisfy requests and percentage of successful log-ins. Grochow performed various checks to determine whether the utility functions over one attribute were independent of the levels of the other attributes (e.g., that the utility of a 5-second response time for simple requests did not depend on the response time for complex requests or availability). Such independence held for eight of the nine systems programmers; the ninth judged log-in availability as less important when response time was slow.

There are several ways in which this decision analysis process could improve decision making. First, by explicitly thinking about the trade-offs among the attributes, the systems analysts may develop a much better understanding of their own preferences, and thus be able to communicate better and to make better decisions about systems. Second, the preference functions of various decision makers can be compared, and the focus of any disagreements highlighted. Finally, knowing the utility function among users of a computer system can be valuable to help the users' supervisor or the time-sharing vendor choose among pricing and service policies to attract customers. In this way, the utility function is substituting for the decision makers, saving time and allowing the consideration of an expanded set of alternatives.

If decision makers are uncertain about what attributes and alternatives are potentially relevant, what levels of attributes to place on the various alternatives, or how much they value the attributes, then decision analysis seems appropriate. In general, however, decision analysis is an expensive and time-consuming task. It usually requires the assistance of a competent professional and, in many ways, the art of aiding decision making can take on an almost clinical or therapeutic air.

WEIGHTED-ADDITIVE MODELS:
A CONSUMER'S GUIDE

Which Weighted-Additive Model to Use?

The choice between descriptive and prescriptive models depends upon the goals of the study: Either you need to describe and predict the decisions made by decision makers, or they need help. Notice that the critical difference between description and prescription lies not in the form of the decision rule or the method of eliciting beliefs and values, but in the way this information gets used. In the Fishbein model, for example, the information is combined in order to predict behavior such as choice among soft drinks. In decision analysis, the information is combined in order to identify what decision makers should choose; indeed, we explicitly are trying to improve upon suboptimal actual behavior.

We should not be lured, however, into an either-or choice between description and prescription. It is often the case that the goal of prescription is facilitated by some preliminary descriptive modeling (to identify issues, and to set the stage to implement prescriptive suggestions). Many descriptive models themselves have been based on prescriptions of optimal performance, or have framed their descriptions as errors and biases by comparing decision makers to prescriptive models.

If the research goal is primarily description of decisions, then it would seem that alternative-based models have a distinct advantage. After all, these methods measure actual decisions or behavior. In general, the research evidence suggests that people have a hard time integrating complex information by themselves; this suggests that one cannot easily predict decisions based on assessments of component attributes (and presumed decision rules), which argues for alternative-based models. If the attributes are very subjective, however, so that attribute evaluations may be quite different from objective values, then it makes sense to assess these subjective judgments in the way typically associated with attribute-based models, although such questions can be used with alternative-based approaches as well.

If the goal is prescription, then the first issue is whether the "correctness" of a decision is defined at the level of an alternative (e.g., higher stock price is better) or at the level of an attribute (e.g., higher gas mileage is better). Prescriptive models are built around what is known, and extrapolated through the use of various theories toward what is not known. Thus, if people understand the quality of attributes better than the quality of holistic alternatives, then an attribute-based model would seem best (and vice versa). A second issue is whether decision makers are more accurate at assessing the parts of problems (attributes and weights) or holistic alternatives. Researchers are just beginning to explore analytic solutions to *when* "divide and conquer" is expected to be a successful strategy to aid decision makers (Ravindar, Kleinmuntz, & Dyer, 1988).

An additional issue is whether the particular approach permits the *testing* of assumptions underlying that approach. Attribute-focused approaches assume a linear representation, but make it difficult to validate this assumption. Alternative-focused approaches can at least question these assumptions by examining nonlinear and configural functions; this may be why alternative-focused models have gotten the lion's share of use. It also seems clear that alternative-focused models are easier to use, although no strong empirical or theoretical arguments appear to underlie this observation.

There is no reason other than cost, however, why attribute-focused and alternative-focused techniques could not be used in conjunction. What is needed is to collect information about attributes, weights, and overall evaluations or outcomes. Such hybrid applications have been used to forecast the demand for new products (Green, 1984). This would seem to be especially appropriate when the goal is to understand decisions as well as to predict them.

Weighted-Additive Models in General

Weighted-additive models are the most common and useful technology we have for predicting choices. Models such as regression and conjoint analysis that use a simple linear representation to predict choices do very well and rarely are surpassed by more complex models. While this success is limited when the attributes are negatively correlated (Einhorn, Kleinmuntz, & Kleinmuntz, 1979; Johnson, Meyer, & Ghose, 1989; Newman, 1977), the useful practical application of these models is widespread.

The predictive ability of weighted-additive models, however, comes at a cost. One of the reasons that linear models are such good predictors is that they can mimic the decisions made by a wide variety of processes. They are sometimes termed "paramorphic models" (Hoffman, 1960), because they can produce the same output without having the same underlying processes as the human decision maker. On the other hand, this is good (especially for prescription and some kinds of prediction) because we don't have to worry much about the exact type of decision process. At the same time, it is also dysfunctional (especially for description) because weighted-additive models don't give us a detailed explanation of how decisions are made. Like aerial photographs, they present a good overall view, but miss some important details of how the information is combined.

There are occasions when these details might be important. For example, if we were designing a computer display of information for stock analysts, then we might want to put the information that analysts look at first at the beginning of the display. While a weighted-additive model might tell us what information is important, it does not tell us how to structure the decision *process*. Providing information in the proper order, for example, may improve accuracy, efficiency, or confidence. Thus, on the whole, weighted-additive models are not very helpful in explaining the details of the decision process, nor in suggesting changes in the process. In the next chapter, we turn to a set of methods whose strengths are complementary to those of weighted-additive models.

NOTES

1. This is similar to the distinction between decompositional versus compositional methods of modeling decisions (Wilkie & Pessimier, 1973).

2. Unfortunately, the published paper does not report the weights. We have assumed a constant equal to 0, and used as illustrative weights the cue validities for the four variables, equivalent to B^2.

3. Unfortunately, the published paper does not give the value for the constant, which we have estimated.

4. More formally, the transformed score, by convention the z, is:

$$z_i = (X_i - X_{\text{Average}}) / (\text{Standard Deviation of } X)$$

SKILL BUILDING

1. Imagine that you work for a manufacturing company in the personnel department. There has been some concern over promotion policies, specifically in regard to minorities and women. It has been alleged in casual discussion that promotion recommendations in particular by male supervisors over 50 years of age are biased. You decide to investigate this issue by building a predictive model of promotion decisions.

   (a) How would you define your research questions?

   (b) Would you create a descriptive or a prescriptive model, or both?

   (c) Would you use alternate-focused or attribute-focused approaches, or some combination?

    (d) What are the alternatives and attributes in this situation?

    (e) Where would you get information from which to build your models?

    (f) How would you deal with characteristics of the supervisor (decision maker)? Are they attributes in the model, or would you build separate models for different supervisor categories?

2. Table 4.3 contains the salaries and offensive statistics for the 1989 Oakland A's and New York Yankees (excluding pitchers). From the data in this table, build a regression model using salaries as the dependent variable, as predicted by a subset of the player performance statistics. Once you have your model, answer the following questions:

    (a) Can you interpret the policy the owners seem to be following? How much is a hit worth, for example, on average?

    (b) How good is the overall model at predicting salaries?

    (c) Were there any particular statistical problems, such as multicollinearity, that you had to deal with in building your model? What did you do?

    (d) Is there anything missing in your model that you would like to include? Are there other factors, outside of the performance variables in Table 4.3, that could influence salaries?

    (e) How does an equal-weight model do compared to your model based on the performance statistics?

Models very much like these are used in the tough business of salary negotiation and litigation in Major League Baseball today. Players have used such models to compare years in which owners have colluded to "normal" years, and to compute damages. Owners have suggested (in the spring of 1990) that players with less than five years of experience be paid by such a formula.

Table 4.3
Major League Player Performance Statistics

Player	Salary	At Bats	Hits	Batting Average	Home Runs	Stolen Bases	Runs Batted In
			New York Yankees				
Balboni	$800,000	300	71	.237	17	0	59
Barfield	$1,300,000	521	122	.234	23	5	67
Blowers	$68,000	38	10	.263	0	0	3
Brookens	$462,500	168	38	.226	4	1	14
Espinoza	$68,000	503	142	.282	0	3	41
Hall	$900,000	361	94	.260	17	0	58
Kelly	$80,000	441	133	.302	9	35	48
Kiefer	$95,000	8	1	.125	0	0	0
Mattingly	$2,200,000	631	191	.303	23	3	113
Meulens	$68,000	28	5	.179	0	0	1
Polonia	$165,000	433	130	.300	3	22	46
Sax	$1,150,000	651	205	.315	5	43	63
Slaught	$650,000	305	88	.251	5	1	38
Velarde	$72,500	100	34	.340	2	0	11
			Oakland A's				
Blankenship	$68,000	125	29	.232	1	5	4
Canseco	$1,600,000	227	61	.269	17	6	57
Gallego	$207,500	357	90	.252	3	7	30
Hassey	$600,000	268	61	.228	5	1	23
Henderson, D.	$850,000	579	145	.250	15	8	80
Henderson, R.	$2,120,000	541	148	.274	12	77	57
Javier	$167,500	310	77	.248	1	12	28
Lansford	$1,325,000	551	185	.336	2	37	52
McGwire	$475,000	490	113	.231	33	1	95
Parker	$1,000,000	553	146	.264	22	0	97
Phillips	$375,000	451	118	.262	4	3	47
Steinbach	$305,000	454	4	.273	7	1	42
Weiss	$190,000	236	55	.233	3	6	21

5

Process Methods

INTRODUCTION

In the last chapter, we suggested that one goal of decision research is *understanding* how decisions are made. To achieve this goal, it would not be sufficient to have an accurate prediction of decisions if that predictive model did not capture the mechanisms within the decision process. Let's take an extreme example: Two loan officers work for a bank. One loan officer accepts 90% of all loan applicants, and the other rejects 90%. We can predict what each loan officer will do based on their past behavior, but we have no understanding of why they behave this way. Process methods seek a deeper understanding of the decision process in order to generate better theories of decision making and to suggest changes in the decision process, thus extrapolating beyond existing descriptive models.

One analogy is that using weighted-additive models is like trying to figure out the workings of a watch from its output. Many different internal mechanisms—which Hoffman (1960) called *paramorphic models*—could produce similar output from the same input. In our analogy, quartz watches are not easily distinguished from mainspring watches by the time they keep. Once we remove the back from the watch, however, we can easily observe what is inside and examine how the mechanism works. This analogy also illustrates when process analysis is inappropriate: if all we need to know is the correct time, then we may not care about what is inside the watch.

In this chapter, we examine several special types of methods and models used to delineate decision processes. We first offer a more complete definition of the cognitive processes of interest, and then describe how process methods are used to gather data and construct process models.

COGNITIVE PROCESSES

The "cognitive revolution" has brought a growing understanding of some basic facts about how people think and reason. Process models of

71

decision making and judgment reflect and depend upon our current knowledge of human information processing. Further, this knowledge guides the use of process methods for the development of models.

There are some central principles of information processing (see Newell & Simon, 1972) that have guided research in cognitive psychology. First, most information processing—especially for high-level tasks such as decision making—is serial. This means that the operations underlying attention, memory, and computation occur one at a time.[1] Even though it may seem that we are working on multiple things at the same time, we do so by alternating among the tasks; no wonder we are easily confused and "lose our train of thought." Second, memory can be thought of as a dual system, with each portion having different capabilities and constraints. There is a relatively small capacity, but easily accessed, short-term memory. Because of its small capacity, there is a bottleneck in attempting to take in all that occurs around us, or to recall relevant information from long-term memory. Backing up short-term memory is a much larger capacity, but much less accessible, long-term memory. Long-term memory is like a library that can store huge amounts of information, but finding the right item can be difficult or impossible without the right "call numbers" or cues.

Characteristics of Process Models

Based upon this framework of cognition, process models characterize the ways in which inputs and outputs are connected by three properties: mediation, time order, and specification of the contents of short-term memory.

Mediation. One of the key properties of process models is that they posit intervening variables between input and output. The goal in process research is to observe these variables. Thus, process models are not only theories of decision making, but also theories about mental events and how to observe them. For example, if we take the linear regression models of judgment in Chapter 4 literally, then we could test whether decision makers seek out information about all the relevant attributes for each alternative, and combine this information into holistic preferences.

Time order. A second property is that process models often suggest a temporal order for events. For example, one common model is that choice among large sets of alternatives consists of two phases that occur in order: an initial screening phase that eliminates objectionable alternatives, and a second trade-off phase where more detailed processing is carried out on a few of the alternatives (Payne, 1976). Such a model makes strong assumptions about the way decision makers will search through information.

Contents of short-term memory. Finally, an important property of process models is that they usually make statements about what a decision maker will and will not know (i.e., the contents of short-term memory) and when they will know it during the course of a decision. For example, if people eliminate bad alternatives early in the decision process, then we could predict that they will remember relatively little about the eliminated alternatives. In contrast, if decision makers make holistic judgments that are compared at the end of the decision process, then the decision makers need not start from scratch in making new decisions about the same alternatives (e.g., what is the second-best choice).

Task Analysis

Process methods rely on a detailed description of the decision or problem called a *task analysis*. It starts with the surface features of the decision by considering the decision maker, the alternatives to be chosen or judgments to be made, the information available to the decision maker, and the circumstances of the decision. If we are studying medical diagnosis, for example, then we should define what diagnoses we are concerned with, make sure that we study people who could reasonably be asked to make such diagnoses, and give these decision makers an appropriate decision task. We could study actual diagnoses as they are being made by real doctors (if possible), or else assemble the kind of lab reports, X rays, photographs, and other materials to create a reason facsimile of the task and give it to volunteer decision makers of the right sort.

The task analysis then goes keep deeper into the processes that are likely to occur as the decision is made. First, decision makers have a representation or mental image of the decision or judgment task, called a *problem space*, formed through the interaction of task information with prior knowledge. The researcher tries to specify the possible states of knowledge or contents of short-term memory that the decision maker might have. Second, the researcher identifies a set of *goals* and subgoals for the decision, which correspond to desired locations or directions in the problem space. Third, the researcher tries to specify a set of *operators* that act on the contents of short-term memory to create new knowledge or—in our terminology—move the decision maker from one point in the problem space to another. In the case of chess players deciding on a move, the problem space consists of possible chess positions that the player envisions; the ultimate goal is to checkmate the opponent with possible subgoals of material and positional advantage; and the operators are procedures to imagine moves and evaluate their consequences. In this way, the chess player searches through the problem space for the best move.

Linear Models as Process Models

A useful exercise is to consider why the linear models discussed in the previous chapter are questionable as process models. First, they make statements that seem implausible given our knowledge of cognition: Combining weights and values through explicit multiplication would simply take too long and quickly overwhelm short-term memory. Second, linear models do not make explicit statements about the time order of events and what is contained in memory (i.e., the problem space and operators). To treat them as process models, we need to add many assumptions about when alternatives are evaluated and when comparisons occur (see Hagarty & Aaker, 1984; Payne, 1976, for examples of such assumptions).

We begin our discussion of ways to collect process-relevant data with the most frequently used process method, verbal protocols. Afterwards, we will turn to a family of process methods that monitor information acquisition, and also briefly mention several other process methods. Finally, we will present our consumer's guide to process methods.

VERBAL PROTOCOLS

Wouldn't it be nice if people could simply tell us what they are thinking as they make decisions? The most common and historically important process-tracing method has been the think-aloud protocol, simply recording what people say when asked to talk aloud as they think. In the 19th century, researchers used the method of introspection, which involved having participants who were highly trained in psychology look inside their own minds and report on their mental processes and their theories of what was going on. This fell into disrepute with the rise of behaviorism in the 1920s, with its emphasis on observable behaviors and avoidance of "mentalistic" explanations.

The verbal protocol method, pioneered by Herbert Simon and Allan Newell, differs from introspection in several key ways, although it did resurrect the procedure of asking participants to think aloud as they did mental tasks. First, people are not asked to speculate about what they are doing, but only to utter what comes to mind as they are thinking. Second, participants are not trained in introspection, although they may be experts in content areas such as chess or medicine. Verbal protocols have been used to study many different aspects of behavior, including problem solving (Newell & Simon, 1972) and problem recognition (Isenberg, 1987), and many different decision tasks, including those of managers (Clarkson, 1962) and consumers (see Bettman, 1979, for a review).

Concurrent Versus Retrospective Reports

It is vital that we draw a distinction between concurrent verbal protocols and the retrospective reports discussed in Chapter 3. This important difference emerges from our theoretical premises about cognition (Ericsson & Simon, 1984). Because of limited attention and the structure of memory, it should be relatively easy to report what one currently is thinking by verbalizing the current contents of short-term memory.

In contrast, when we ask people how they have made decisions *after* they have finished, very little information about the decision remains in short-term memory. It is also likely that very little information has been transferred to long-term memory. As a result, retrospective reports are incomplete, and subject to fabrication and reconstruction ("That is how I must have done it . . ."). The series of studies by Nisbett and Wilson (1977) is a particularly good demonstration of the hazards of retrospective reports. Thus, our model of cognition guides our data collection: What can be obtained most accurately from verbal protocols is an ongoing report of the changing contents of short-term memory.

Collecting Verbal Protocols

The theory of protocol generation also tells us how to collect concurrent protocols. It is important—according to Ericsson and Simon (1984)—not to ask a decision maker for specific types of information, particularly if that information normally would not be salient while doing the task. This prohibition recognizes that such requests can cause the decision makers to alter their attention or to try to fulfill the request, thus changing the underlying process and invalidating the protocol.

For example, we might be tempted to ask the decision makers to report how they weight the attributes in a choice task, while they are in the midst of the task (or a series of decisions). Such instructions, however, run the risk of changing their strategies: Decision makers who would normally ignore an attribute might now attend to it because the questioning suggests they should "weight attributes." There is also an additional risk of having them fabricate their own theories of how they *think* they decided. Thus, protocol instructions should not ask for explanations, but simply ask participants to talk aloud, saying whatever comes to mind.

One reasonable set of instructions comes from the classic book by Ericsson and Simon (1984):

> In this experiment we are interested in what you say to yourself as you perform some tasks that we give you. In order to do this we will ask you to TALK ALOUD as you work on the problems. What I mean by talk aloud is that I want you to say out loud everything that you say to yourself silently. Just act as if you are alone in the room speaking to yourself. If you are silent for any length of time I will remind you to keep talking aloud. Do you understand what I want you to do? (p. 376)

Russo, Johnson and Stephens (1989) have suggested that the instructions also emphasize the option of remaining silent if the cognitive demands of the current primary task—making a decision—do not allow a decision maker to talk aloud. Long silences, however, may also indicate that the decision maker has stopped talking simply because talking aloud is inconvenient and unnatural. The researcher can prompt the decision maker with neutral, nondirective statements, such as "What are you thinking now?" or "Please remember to talk aloud."

Prior practice on an unrelated task can help decision makers become more comfortable with verbalizing their thoughts. Ericsson and Simon (1984) suggest using a warm-up task, such as mental multiplication (multiply 24 times 34) or anagrams (unscramble NPEPHA into HAPPEN). Verbal protocols are usually recorded with an unobtrusive tape recorder.

Finally, the researcher must resist the occasional temptation to interact with participants in a less formal manner. Recording verbal protocols is not an interview, and asking for explanations represents a major threat to the validity of protocol generation. The assumption is that anything the researcher does to suggest values or strategies or to encourage some behavior could affect the subject's decisions and distort the observations. This is in direct contrast to the way informal methods typically encourage exchanges and probing at all times, and treat participants more as collaborators.

The critical issues are how sensitive participants are to the researcher's requests and probes, how conscious and well-practiced is the decision process (so that people can report accurately and be uninfluenced by the probing), and how sensitive researchers are to possible threats to validity. One possible reconciliation of these approaches is to collect verbal protocols *during* the task and to conduct a probing interview *after* the protocols are collected, on subsequent decisions, or on a different group of decision makers.

Protocol Analysis

Gathering protocol data may seem relatively easy, as long as the conditions for valid verbal reports are met. This is just the first step, however, of the long and arduous process of analyzing the reports. The depth of analysis depends in large part on how well the task is known and the purposes for doing the analysis. We will distinguish among three types of analysis: (1) informal exploratory analysis, (2) content analysis of statement frequencies, and (3) construction of formal simulation models.

Exploratory analysis. Exploratory analysis often starts and stops with reading the transcribed protocols. Such informal analysis is usually employed when there is only limited knowledge about the task, how it is done, and what information is used by the decision maker. It is typical to focus on the "best" protocols, that is, the participants who have verbalized thoroughly. One frequent application uses protocols to "debug" questionnaires prior to administration in a large survey: A small sample of people is asked to complete the questionnaire, talking aloud while doing so. The resulting protocols are examined for evidence that the questionnaire is vague or confusing. Similarly, in marketing applications, protocols are used to identify attributes from which the researcher then constructs hypothetical products for conjoint analysis (see Chapter 6) or other structured methods.

Even a simple reading of a series of protocols provides considerable information, regardless of whether one will proceed with expensive coding. It is possible to observe how decision makers break up the decision task into concepts or attributes, which of these seem important or salient, the order in which attributes are noticed, how these considerations are combined into judgments and decisions, and whether there are differences across decision makers or decision instances.

Table 5.1 provides an excerpt from the verbal protocol of an experienced shoplifter walking through a retail store (Weaver & Carroll, 1985). It is instructive, for example, to list the attributes of the store and individual items that are expressed, the motivations that are verbalized, and the way the shoplifter can imagine alternative actions. In this way,

Table 5.1

Shoplifter Verbal Protocol Excerpt

So moving on, moving on over to the hardware department I think sounds pretty good; might be something there I could use. 'Cause I don't really have very many tools, and every now and then, I like to make little tinkering repairs and so, it might be a nice idea to check it out here, see what you could do. . . . Security in the store looks pretty good so far, they've got a lot of people standing around, but, uh, the layout of the store looks like you could hide behind counters, put something in a pocket, um, rather easily there doesn't look like there's any overhead mirrors or remote security systems. OK, here we go, we're getting down close to the hardware department. Let's see what all they got. Doesn't look like it's very well stocked at all. In fact, it's terrible. Um, bug spray, batteries. Batteries, of course, would be easy to take out. Um, although there is somebody standing here, so I have to be careful, move rather slowly, just kind of browse around a little bit. . . . Glass cutters, wrenches. The packaging here would make lifting fairly easily if you had a nice big coat, in the wintertime, with kind of large pockets. Everything is flat, um, visibility from other departments is poor. Oh, this this would be easy to lift. This would be really easy to lift. You could take any one of these things off the rack. Now, of course, these are small items, but then, a lot of times, tool needs are for small items, I mean, here's a six-inch adjustable wrench, um, fit into my pocket fairly easily, um, the utility knife, padlock, um, generally useful items you could put 'em in right away, fuses, switches, um, small extension cords. It, this would be really easy to lift in here. Um, now some of the other bigger items, like light bulbs and timers and things, those wouldn't go over, but um, if I needed something, I'd probably pick it out from up here, that would be relatively simple.

---

informal analysis of the protocols can enhance our understanding of the decision process and offer hypotheses for further analysis.

Content analysis. Content analysis of protocols requires an added degree of structure and effort. In order to portray more carefully the processes captured in the protocol, we *categorize* the statements to reflect different kinds of mental events. This process begins with a careful analysis of the task, leading to the construction of a coding scheme representing the mental operations that we believe might be used to make a decision (see Bettman & Park, 1980, for an extensive example of a coding scheme for consumer choice; and Beihal & Charkravarti, 1982, for a discussion of its application and limitations).

Before coding begins, there is the preliminary task of transcription in which streams of tape-recorded statements are *segmented* into units. These units are judged to reflect single complete thoughts (Newell & Simon, 1972). Pauses between phrases ("Umm . . . ") are one guide that can be used to segment the protocol. One segmented protocol, taken

Table 5.2

A Coded Verbal Protocol of Apartment Search

Statement	Code
Let's just see what the rents are in all the apartments first.	GOAL
The rent of A is $140.	READ(A, Rent)
The rent of B is $110.	READ(B, Rent)
The rent of C is $170.	READ(C, Rent)
Um, $170 is too much	ELIMINATE(C)
(. . .)	
I'm going to look at landlord attitude.	GOAL
In H it's Fair.	READ (H, Landlord Attitude)
(. . .)	

(Adapted from Payne et al., 1978, pp. 24-25)

from an example we will describe in depth, is given in Table 5.2. It contains statements from a student deciding among several hypothetical apartments (labeled A through H), each described by attributes such as rent, number of rooms, and location.

Table 5.2 includes some of the codes used in a study of apartment selection (Payne, 1976). The specific task was to select information about hypothetical apartments from a set of envelopes arrayed in rows and columns by alternative and attribute, and to select the preferred apartment. A task analysis of possible choice strategies suggested that several distinct mental operations might be performed: information has to be READ, might be COMPARED, and alternatives could be ELIMINATED. Thus, the initial coding scheme reflects a best guess about what processing might occur during the task. The coding scheme is typically revised as coders note which codes are difficult to use, too broad or overlapping, or as new categories of statements are induced from the protocols.

Our next goal is to categorize each of the statements in the protocol into one coding category or another. In Table 5.2, the second statement would be categorized as a "read," because it simply describes a piece of information about the apartments and reflects no other cognitive processing. To help limit possible biases, the process of coding is usually done by coders who did not know the details of the research hypotheses, but are working with a set of *coding rules* prepared by the researchers. At least two different coders work independently to see if there is sufficient agreement in assigning the statements into categories.

When a coding scheme is sufficiently detailed, and the coders are sufficiently trained, agreement can be quite high. It is commonplace for statements to be coded into the same categories about 90% of the time by two independent coders. Such agreement demonstrates that the categories have an explicit, communicable existence apart from the judgments of the researchers. Note the contrast to informal methods, which typically rely on the subjective understandings of the researcher all the way to the final report.

Armed with the results of our coding, we can extend our understanding of the underlying processes. For example, in the study of apartment choice illustrated in Table 5.2, Payne (1976) considered four alternative decision models. One of them, additive utility (the linear models of Chapter 4), suggests that people explicitly weight each of the attributes of the available apartments. Very few of the protocols, however, contained explicit weightings. Instead, there were many statements consistent with an elimination-by-aspect strategy (Tversky, 1972) that ruled out apartments failing to meet apparent cutoffs (e.g., too expensive, too far from campus). Thus, by examining the frequencies of various kinds of statements, we can add support for some models and lessen our belief in others.

It is also informative to examine the relationships among various statement types, compare frequencies of codes during time periods of the protocol (e.g., early, middle, and late portions), or compare frequencies under variations in tasks, situations, and decision makers. For example, Weaver and Carroll (1985) examined the differences between experienced and novice shoplifters. They found that they could identify items that had received an explicit comment about "taking" or "not taking" the items, and that these could be related to the presence of facilitators (factors conducive to shoplifting) and deterrents (factors that prevent shoplifting). Novices always mentioned one facilitator and no deterrents when they decided to take an item; the presence of a single deterrent was sufficient to stop novices from concluding they would take the item. In contrast, when experts mentioned a deterrent, it was often followed by mention of a facilitator allowing the deterrent to be discounted or outweighed, and an expressed willingness to shoplift. In Table 5.1, for example, the experienced shoplifter notes as a deterrent that security is "pretty good . . . a lot of people standing around" but follows with the facilitator that "you could hide behind counters, put something in a pocket, um, rather easily."

Explicit models. As our understanding of the decision process develops, we can build explicit models of the task with detailed tests of their implications. A first step in this type of analysis is to construct a *problem space* that specifies the possible knowledge that decision makers can acquire during the task, along with a set of goals and subgoals for that task. We can combine this with a set of operators developed from the coding scheme that act on the knowledge that is present, and create new knowledge. An example would be the operator COMPARE, which examines two alternatives and produces the information that one is better than the other on an attribute. A decision process can then be described as a series of operators that are used to move through the problem space until a goal is reached (e.g., knowing which apartment to choose). Clearly, such a level of analysis requires an in-depth understanding of the task.

Given this detailed understanding of the operators and problem space, the codes in the verbal protocol can be represented as a *problem behavior graph* or flowchart that shows the sequence in which operations occur, and the information flowing in and out of each operation. A detailed theory of how people are thought to behave in a task can produce a similar (hypothetical) trace of the operations in the same task. A comparison between the problem behavior graphs from the protocols and those from the theoretical model provide strong tests of the descriptive validity of the models.

A natural next step is to express the theory in the form of a *computer simulation* rather than a series of verbal propositions. The advantage of the computer simulation is that it forces a level of specificity seldom reached in others ways. The propositions built into the computer simulation can be tested for consistency and explored for implications by running the program. After running the program, traces of the intermediate steps in computer processing can be compared to the traces made by actual decision makers as represented in problem behavior graphs. Table 5.3 provides such a trace of the computer simulation of apartment choice. (Interested readers should refer to Newell & Simon, 1972; and Ericsson & Simon, 1984).

As you can tell, protocol analysis requires significant investment of time and resources. There is the labor of gathering and transcribing protocols, a significant intellectual effort to build a careful coding scheme or a complete task analysis before analyzing the data, and a lengthy period of coding and analyzing the results. The cost of protocol analysis prevents

Table 5.3
Protocol and Model Trace

Protocol	Model Trace
Let's see what the rents are in all the apartments first.	I WILL NOW LOOK AT THE RENT OF EACH ALTERNATIVE.
The rent of A is $140.	THE RENT OF A IS $140.
The rent of B is $110.	THE RENT OF B IS $110.
The rent of C is $170.	THE RENT OF C IS $170.
(. . .)	
Um, $170 is too much.	ALTERNATIVE C ELIMINATED.
But, if the other ones aren't good, I'll look at them later.	ALTERNATIVE E ELIMINATED.
But right now I'll look at the other ones.	ALTERNATIVE F ELIMINATED.
	ALTERNATIVE G ELIMINATED.
(. . .)	
I'm going to look at landlord attitude.	I WILL NOW LOOK AT THE LANDLORD OF EACH ALTERNATIVE.
In H it's fair.	THE LANDLORD OF A IS GOOD.
In D it's poor.	THE LANDLORD OF B IS FAIR.
In B it's fair, and	THE LANDLORD OF D IS POOR.
in A it's good.	THE LANDLORD OF H IS FAIR.
So, one of them . . . is poor.	ALTERNATIVE D ELIMINATED.
So that's important to me.	ALTERNATIVE I ELIMINATED.
(. . .)	ALTERNATIVE K ELIMINATED.
So, I'm not going to live any place where it's poor.	ALTERNATIVE L ELIMINATED.
(. . .)	
Oh, J and H have better kitchen facilities than A and B.	ALTERNATIVE A ELIMINATED.
Everything else about the same.	ALTERNATIVE B ELIMINATED.
So eliminate those two.	SINCE I'VE ONLY GOT TWO ALTERNATIVES I WILL APPLY A
And, decide between these two.	COMPENSATORY DECISION PROCESS.
	THE CHOICE IS BETWEEN H AND J.
(. . .)	
Landlord attitude in J is better than in H.	LET'S SEE ON LANDLORD. J IS BETTER.
(. . .)	
In J the rooms are larger.	LET'S SEE ON SIZE.
So, I guess, J will be better.	J IS BETTER.
	I CHOOSE ALTERNATIVE J.

(Adapted from Payne et al., 1978, pp. 24-25)

it from being applied to large samples of decision makers, or even to large numbers of decision problems. Typical studies include 12 or fewer subjects, and few decision problems; some classic studies concern the behavior of a single subject on a single problem.

Sometimes, it is clearly not worth the effort to do protocol analysis. If the goal is to predict decisions, then developing some form of weighted-additive model is likely to be more cost-effective (Einhorn, Kleinmuntz, & Kleinmuntz, 1979). If there is a need to reach a process-level understanding of decisions, then the researchers must assess the suitability of the decision task for protocols, and their willingness to pay the costs. Tasks that have been profitably studied seem to have been: (1) fairly short; (2) repetitive; (3) not so highly structured that people simply read materials in order; (4) not so unstructured that responses are idiosyncratic and hard to code; and (5) verbally processed, that is, not based on nonverbal or overlearned skills that are inaccessible to consciousness (imagine verbal protocols of table tennis!).

SEARCH METHODS

Protocol analysis resembles eavesdropping: We listen, somewhat surreptitiously, to the conversations that decision makers have with themselves as they make choices and judgments. In contrast, methods that observe information acquisitions are voyeuristic, because they involve watching people as they make decisions.

The core of search methods—as we will call them—is monitoring the physical behaviors used to acquire information as people make decisions. By observing what information is considered and the order in which it is acquired, we hope to infer the cognitive processes underlying the decisions.

When making decisions, one can access two sources of information: (1) the external environment, and (2) internal memory. In most decision tasks, externally available information plays a vital role, and it is here that search methods can be most useful. Because the capacity of short-term memory is limited, a decision maker often will depend upon the presence of information in the external environment. To the extent that information acquisition is easy, then the link between acquisition and use will be strong, and information acquisitions will be a good reflection of the ongoing decision process.

Monitoring Devices

Search methods are better understood if we examine how we can monitor information acquisition. Quite a range of possibilities exist, from high-tech to mundane.

Eye-movement monitoring. At the high-technology end are devices that monitor decision makers' eye movements as they examine displays of information. Sensory physiologists know that the eye acquires detailed information such as text from the fovea, a narrow area near the center of the field of view. Furthermore, the eye does not see much while performing saccades (the quick, ballistic motions from one spot to another). Therefore, recording the location and duration of the pauses between moves—the *eye fixations*—allows us to monitor the information that is being read for the decisions.

The level of detail provided by eye-movement recording is quite high, and it is possible to covertly monitor eye fixations. Eye-movement monitors, however, are expensive, technically complicated, and unlikely to be employed by readers of this book.

Manual information display. At the low-technology extreme are information display boards: physical arrays in which the information about the alternatives and their attributes is concealed in envelopes with labels along the rows and columns representing alternatives and attributes. To retrieve a piece of information, the decision maker must pick up the corresponding card and turn it over, usually returning it to its envelope after reading. The researcher usually records manually the order of acquisition, noting the rows and columns of the cards examined.

Other variations of manual information acquisition are possible. For example, Bennett and Wright (1984) used a set of photographs of potential burglary targets. They started by handing experienced burglars a photo of the front of a house, and then permitted them to request additional photos in an unstructured way. The burglar might say, "What does it look like from the rear?" or "Show me the neighbor's house on the right." The researcher would then interpret this request and provide an appropriate photo; between 26 and 36 photos were available for each of five houses. Burglars requested about four additional photos on average.

Computers. In between the high- and low-technology extremes are recent developments that employ computers to present information displays to decision makers. The requests for information are made using a variety of input and pointing devices including keyboards, trackballs

(Payne & Braunstein, 1978), joysticks, light pens (Jacoby, Jaccard, Kuss, Troutman, & Mazursky, 1985), and mice (Johnson, Mayer, & Ghose, 1989). These systems have the advantage of automatically recording with high accuracy the pattern and duration of information acquisition and the resultant judgments or decisions. Because these devices make the recording of process data easier, we expect them to have a major impact in encouraging process-tracing research.

Finally, we should note that as computerized decision support becomes more commonplace, it becomes more and more practical to build into the workplace a capability to monitor information acquisition as part of everyday life. For example, we might study someone who searches a computer data base to generate alternatives by recording the pattern of queries issued. As computerized tools become a bigger part of everyday life, opportunities for such "data traps" (Keen & Scott-Morton, 1978) will grow (see Chapter 8 for a discussion of these possibilities).

An Example: Apartment Hunting

Although we have described the various methods that can be used to collect a record of the information examined by decision makers, we have not been very explicit about how these data are analyzed. Let us consider the apartment choice example used previously in our discussion of verbal protocols.

The choice models considered by Payne (1976) have very different implications for how information will be searched. The additive utility model (which looks much like the linear models of Chapter 4) suggests that information is searched *within an alternative*, in order to compute a utility score for that alternative before moving on to the next alternative. Furthermore, this reasoning suggests that the same attributes are examined for every alternative.

Elimination by aspects, on the other hand, suggests that a decision maker might look at the value of all the alternatives for one attribute before moving on to the next attribute. This is called a *dimensional* search strategy. If an alternative is eliminated, then no further information will be searched with regard to that alternative. As a result, we should see more information acquired about the alternatives that remain under consideration—particularly for the alternative eventually chosen—than for those quickly eliminated.

Search data are usually analyzed by constructing simple *indices* of search patterns. For example, the standard deviation of the number of items searched across alternatives would provide an index of how unevenly alternatives were scanned. The proportion of *transitions* (the movements from one item to the next) that are within-alternative/across-attribute can be compared to the proportion that are across-alternative/within-attribute.

The patterns in Payne's study were very similar to those predicted by an elimination-by-aspects strategy: Most subjects used dimensional search strategies, and examined different amounts of information across alternatives. Over 91% of the time, the chosen alternative was searched as much or more than any other (Russo, 1978, had a similar result using eye fixations; and Johnson & Meyer, 1984, had similar results using verbal protocols). Both of these trends were more pronounced for decisions with more alternatives or attributes. Thus, the search data suggested that subjects used elimination strategies, particularly when the decision task was more complex.

OTHER PROCESS METHODS

In our limited review, we cannot detail other important and interesting alternatives for process-tracing research. Yet the possible techniques are limited only by the information and resourcefulness of the researcher. By careful application of the ideas we have presented in this section, an interesting process method unique to the research situation can often be devised. As an example of a clever way to monitor information acquisition, Russo (1978) discussed television cameras positioned behind one-way mirrors in simulated supermarkets to observe how long people looked at a new type of nutritional labeling.

Monitoring Communications

The monitoring of group conversations or organizational messages also provides a trace of processes at individual and group levels. At an individual level, messages received are comparable to information acquisitions, and messages sent are like verbal protocols. At the group level, observations of communications are much like verbal protocols, allowing us to listen in on the group decision process. For example, content analysis of electronic mail has been used to study the frequency of highly emotional messages in real organizations, which Kiesler, Siegel, and McGuire (1984) refer to as "flaming." Tape recordings of mock jury deliberations have been used to create theories of jury decision making, and to evaluate the impact of different decision rules on verdicts and deliberation quality (Hastie, Penrod, & Pennington, 1983).

Recall Techniques

If verbal protocols resemble eavesdropping, and monitoring search and communication are voyeuristic, then recall techniques resemble archaeology—trying to figure out what happened in the past by looking at what remains in the present storehouse of memory. Researchers use various methods borrowed from cognitive psychology to assess memory, and presume that the current contents of memory enable inferences about the focus of attention during decisions. For example, elimination by aspects suggests that people will not look at information about bad alternatives; thus, we can predict poor recall for rejected alternatives. Memory following consumer decisions shows exactly this pattern (Beihal & Charkravarti, 1982; Johnson & Russo, 1984).

Chronometric Techniques

Chronometric techniques measure the amount of time that it takes to perform decision tasks. The basic logic is simple: If we believe that a decision process consists of steps, then we can specify the amount of time it should take to complete tasks of varying complexity (number and type of processing steps).

For example, people who use an additive utility strategy must execute the same process—of reading information, combining it with the attribute importance weights, and developing an overall evaluation—for every alternative. Thus, we would predict that adding alternatives should have a linear effect on decision time: Each new alternative should cause the same increase in decision processes and, therefore, decision time. Onken, Hastie, and Revelle (1985) tested this model by looking at the total amount of time that it took students to choose apartments for decisions with different numbers of alternatives and attributes. They found that decision time did not increase linearly, but rather that the increase slowed down as the number of alternatives increased; for some subjects, bigger decision problems even resulted in shorter latencies. Onken, Hastie, and Revelle took this as evidence that subjects switched to simplifying strategies such as elimination by aspects, a notion consistent with Payne's (1976) results.

PROCESS METHODS: A CONSUMER'S GUIDE

As the impact of the cognitive revolution grows, it seems clear that we will see increased application of process methods in decision making. Along with more sophisticated ideas about cognition, the successful application of process-tracing techniques requires a more complete understanding of the cognitive processes underlying the decisions observed. Thus, theory and method develop together.

Is This Really Necessary?

Process techniques (in comparison to the development of weighted-additive models in Chapter 4) are labor intensive, requiring extensive effort on the part of the person studying the decision process and/or special equipment. The few existing comparisons between process and weighted-additive models show them to be about equal in predicting the outcome of choices (Einhorn, Kleinmuntz, & Kleinmuntz, 1979).

Then why construct process models? Primarily because they increase our understanding of the decision process in ways that weighted-additive models usually do not. The goal of process models is to increase the number of variables that can be examined by a model of decision making. In addition to outcome variables such as final choices or judgments, process analysis extends to the verbal utterances and information search conducted by decision makers. By using such data, process models provide additional powerful tools for identifying, developing, and selecting alternative models of decision making.

Choosing Among Process Techniques

As we have suggested throughout this chapter, process techniques are oriented toward different aspects of decision behavior. Researchers should approach a project by trying to construct a task analysis, and then thinking carefully about how the elements of the task analysis match up against the strengths and weaknesses of various process techniques.

For decision tasks in which the major operations include accessing information in memory and manipulating information with operators that can be reported on (e.g., mental arithmetic), verbal protocols would seem to be a good choice. Information acquisition techniques would not match the nature of the task, because there are few external signs of mental activity. Verbal protocols would also be useful if information is accessed externally, but we cannot specify the bits and pieces ahead of time (as in the case of a shoplifter walking through a store and looking around). If the task required a high-speed visual search through information with overlearned strategies that were no longer accessible to verbal report (for example, playing a video arcade game), then we might try eye-movement recording, video recording, and possibly playing these event records back to the subjects for their commentary after the fact. (For a discussion of prompted protocols, see Russo & Dosher, 1983.) Information acquisition techniques are most useful when a manageable amount of specific external information is being accessed.

The question of *which* process technique to use is in some ways misleading; it assumes that a choice between methods *must* be made. Several authors (Payne, Braunstein, & Carroll, 1978; Russo, 1978), however, suggest that multiple methods are best. Weaknesses in one method can be complemented by the strengths of another. For example, one problem with eye-movement recording is identifying exactly what thinking lies behind patterns of eye movements. Verbal protocols can help to identify what underlies certain acquisition patterns. At the same time, eye fixations can help validate a process detected using protocols, because they offer relatively uncensored records of cognition. In our example of apartment choice, the use of verbal protocols and search methods provided considerably more insight than did either method by itself.

This call for multiple-method research can be extended to include combinations of weighted-additive and process methods as well. Ideally, they should complement one another reasonably well. Weighted-additive models can be produced at low cost; process-tracing techniques uncover more of the underlying process. As the technology for process models becomes less forbidding, the frequency of such applications should grow.

NOTE

1. Lower level cognitive tasks, such as identifying an object, are essentially parallel. Future work may both drastically alter the validity of the assumption that higher level tasks are serial, and provide new methods and models of parallelism.

SKILL BUILDING

1. We suggest that you become very self-conscious. Identify a decision or judgment that you have to make in the next day or so; it might involve going to a movie, out to dinner, buying a gift, or whatever. Get a small tape recorder and collect your own verbal protocol from this decision.

    (a) Look at the protocol as an indicator of a weighted-additive model. What were your alternatives? What attributes mattered? What decision rule (weights) was adopted?

    (b) Construct a task analysis. Break up the protocol into separate statements. What did you know at each stage of the decision, what were your goals, and what operators or mental steps did you take to move along to a decision? This is really a content analysis of the protocol.

    (c) Construct a problem behavior graph, representing your state of knowledge at each point in time, and the operators that acted on each point.

    (d) Did the protocol analysis add anything to your understanding of the decision? Are the strategies you used—or the operators you used—very different from the weighted-additive models of Chapter 4, or quite consistent with them?

2. Let's take a situation similar to one in Chapter 4. Your company is interested in understanding more about its internal promotion decisions. Assume that you can get a great deal of cooperation from decision makers and managers.

    (a) What process-tracing techniques will seem useful in this situation? What issues will you consider in trying to decide whether to use any process methods and, if so, which ones?

    (b) What would you do to carry out the study?

    (c) How would you deal with the resulting data? Many researchers fail to realize the volume of (sometimes messy) data that process methods can generate. Think seriously about what you need, what you will get, and what you can do.

6

Creating Controlled Tasks

INTRODUCTION

There are research situations in which the use of realistic materials is very inefficient or ineffective. For example, in our stock price prediction task, many of the available characteristics of stocks co-vary strongly: last year's earnings are usually related to last year's sales, price-earnings ratio, dividends, and so forth. If we try to model stock analysts' price predictions, we find that several combinations of stock characteristics do about as well (i.e., they are paramorphic models). In essence, to know whether investment experts are using earnings or sales in their judgments of price changes, we must rely on the very few stocks that have atypical combinations of characteristics: high earnings with low sales, or low earnings despite high sales. Due to high correlations among earnings and sales (multicollinearity), there may be so few stocks of these types that we cannot distinguish among several variations of the model, especially when the data contain substantial unpredictable components (random noise).

In Chapter 5 we suggested process-tracing methods as one way to add information about decision making. Thus, if decision makers generally look at information about earnings but not about sales, or make comments suggesting that their calculations or judgments are based on earnings, then this would provide evidence about which characteristics of stocks are important, and which models are more descriptively accurate.

A second way to add information is to ask decision makers to judge a series of stocks that contain more of the atypical, but highly informative, instances. Slovic (1969) did exactly this by creating hypothetical stocks using a factorial design (all possible combinations of several stock characteristics). Such a design offers very efficient *controlled comparisons* that separate the individual and configural effects of the various cues or characteristics. What is given up, however, is that decision makers will be evaluating an unusual (and perhaps peculiar) set of stocks.

Hypothetical, highly controlled decision situations are useful for at least two other reasons: They permit researchers to present to decision makers situations or alternatives that do not currently exist, and to develop and test theories of decision making. A typical example of the former is the marketer introducing a new product with features consumers have never seen—such as a car with four-wheel steering, or a sweet, low-calorie dessert. Evaluating new product concepts would be difficult indeed if companies actually had to manufacture each new product idea and introduce it to see if the product could be a success. A typical example of theory testing is to create an explicit comparison between experimental conditions (such as decision makers asked to bid for items versus other decision makers asked to choose among the same items).

This chapter focuses on techniques for creating informative events that permit controlled comparisons. Control means that the comparisons are designed in such a way that there are few opportunities for other factors to intrude into the research and create confounding effects. Thus, researchers need not be content to look for informative events in the world around them; subtle issues are not always illuminated by mundane events. It may take a special set of circumstances—constructed by the researcher—to permit precise comparisons of specific events in order to advance knowledge.

We will first look more closely at situations in which attributes are factorially varied by using hypothetical alternatives. Second, we will examine research in which the existence of an explicit theory permits the construction of very precise questions that test the theory. Third, we will examine situations in which the attributes of decision tasks are varied in controlled experiments.

HYPOTHETICAL ALTERNATIVES

Research with hypothetical alternatives requires some preliminary knowledge of the alternatives and attributes present in typical decisions. From prior research examining naturalistic decisions, discussions with experts, or theories that specify the components of the decision, the researcher must construct decision stimuli that address the research questions, permit controlled comparisons, and engage the knowledge and motivation of the respondent decision makers.

Because the goals and logic of research with hypothetical alternatives are similar to those of weighted-additive models (discussed in Chapter 4), they do not need further introduction. The analysis is in fact very similar, with only a change in how the input (the observed preferences) is obtained. To make this clearer, we will present specific research issues through a concrete example.

An Example: Medical Diagnosis of Ulcer Malignancy

Hoffman, Slovic, and Rorer (1968) wondered whether expert decision makers really use information in nonlinear or configural ways, an issue discussed at length in Chapter 4. They chose to study the diagnosis of malignancy of gastric ulcers by radiologists. This is a diagnostic task in which medical experts report using configural patterns of cues (characteristics of ulcers). The method Hoffman, Slovic, and Rorer used allowed them to separate the linear from the configural effects of the cues by using hypothetical stimuli in a factorial design.

The researchers first consulted with a gastroenterologist to identify the characteristics of ulcers that are used in this diagnosis. There were seven characteristics or signs, such as whether the ulcer contour is regular (yes or no), located on the greater curvature (yes or no), and so forth. Since each sign could be present or absent, there were 2^7 or 128 possible combinations of signs. A competent gastroenterologist examined all possible combinations, and declared 32 of them to be meaningless: all 32 involved impossible pairings of two particular signs. These two signs were recombined into a single three-level sign. The remaining 96 profiles were considered plausible.

Six practicing radiologists and three radiologists-in-training were presented with all 96 cases twice, in random order, and asked to rate them on a 7-point scale from 1 (definitely benign) to 7 (definitely malignant). By presenting the cases twice, the researchers could calculate the reliability of each decision-maker, and calculate within-subject error terms for each physician. The data were analyzed using separate analyses of variance (ANOVA) for each decision maker, and one large ANOVA using the radiologists as another factor.

There were several interesting results. First, there was only a moderate degree of agreement among the radiologists. The median correlation between pairs of radiologists, computed across the cases, was .38. Even after removing the three most unreliable radiologists (assuming they are the ones in training, with reliability computed as the correlation between the two replications of the same cases), the median correlation was only .52. (This gives substantial value to "second opinions"!) Second, main effects of the six signs accounted for an average of over 70% of the variance in radiologists' judgments, whereas the total of all interactions (57 are possible: 15 two-way, 20 three-way, etc.) accounted for about 7%; the largest interaction for any of the nine radiologists accounted for only 3% of the variance. In other words, a linear model could do an adequate job of accounting for the radiologists' judgments. There were a few two-way and three-way interactions, however, that were reliable for the radiologists as a group. Third, the nine radiologists differed significantly in the way they used the signs, which indicates that some of the disagreement among radiologists was due to individually different diagnostic rules.

Related Techniques

There are several other techniques using hypothetical stimuli that are widely used. Two of these will be discussed here: information integration theory and conjoint analysis.

Information Integration Theory. Information integration theory (Anderson, 1981) proposes that cues in a decision task are transformed into *scale values* on a *response function* which are integrated in ways that often follow simple mathematical formulas called *cognitive algebras*, such as the weighted averaging rule prevalent in Chapter 4 and the multiplicative rule in expected utility theory.

Anderson (1981) developed a special research design and measurement technique called *functional measurement* that presents factorially designed combinations of cues to decision makers, and examines integration rules through analysis of variance. The technique goes beyond factorial designs by including presentation of single cues to decision makers. For example, a study of dating choice as a function of a photograph and an expressed probability of accepting a date provided factorial combinations of photos and probabilities, and also asked respondents to respond to photos alone (Shanteau & Nagy, 1976).

Examination of the results can distinguish among various integration rules such as adding, averaging, multiplication, and so forth. The advantage of analysis of variance is that its results are *scale-free*, that is, it does not require any assumptions about the scaling of the cues. Typically, some monotone transformation of the cues as values on the response scale produces a well-behaved integration function. As a result, functional measurement is simultaneously examining valuation, integration, and response functions.

A significant advantage of functional measurement is that it separates the range of an attribute, represented in the scale values, from how much weight it receives from the decision maker. Thus, one attribute could have a wide range of values, yet still be given a lower weight than a second attribute with a narrower range of values. The focus of information integration is on identifying the kind of decision rule employed, and Anderson (1981) seeks to uncover a large variety of such cognitive algebras. In this sense, functional measurement tests the combination rules that most weighted-additive models (see Chapter 4) simply assume.

Conjoint Analysis. One of the most popular market research techniques is called conjoint analysis (Green 1984; Green & Wind, 1975). Cattin and Wittick (1982) conducted a survey of marketers that showed literally hundreds of applications for this technique. While its origins are quite different from the analysis of variance approach, it is closely related in practice. This is best illustrated with a concrete example.

Imagine that a marketer is designing a new portable computer. There are many different possible designs, and the marketer would like to know how much consumers value each of these design attributes. For example, how do consumers value battery life compared to carrying weight?

Conjoint analysis begins by describing all the attributes that are relevant for decision makers, such as cost, memory, disk storage, brand name, and so forth. If these attributes are not immediately apparent, interviews with consumers (see Chapter 3) might be used. The researcher then picks at least two realistic levels on each attributes—for example, prices of $1,500 and $2,500. If the attribute is important or the researcher expects different levels of the attribute to have very different effects, more than two levels may be selected. The chosen levels of each attribute are combined to create hypothetical stimuli; however, in some realistic settings, there may be too many possible combinations to assess easily. A product with seven attributes, each having three levels (not an unrealistic number for a complex product like a computer), would have 3^7 or 2187 total possibilities! To get around this, conjoint analysis makes the assumption that linear models of decision making usually need only main effects to account for preferences (see Chapter 4). By assuming that certain combinations of stimuli (interactions in ANOVA) are unimportant, a *fractional factorial* design (Cochran & Cox, 1957) can be used to cut down the number of hypothetical stimuli: our 2187 hypothetical products could be reduced to as few as 81 or even 27!

Finding the right design for a decision problem, however, can be tricky. In the past, consultants provided expertise in experimental design. More recently, several software packages have appeared that help manage entire projects, from designing experiments through gathering data to providing analysis. For a basic discussion of the many variants of conjoint analysis and research issues, see Green, Helsen, and Shandler (1988).

THE QUESTION-ANSWERING TECHNIQUE

A special variant of using controlled tasks has been pioneered by Daniel Kahneman and Amos Tversky. Their work can be characterized as building creative theories from simple (but elegant) questions. We will present their approach through some examples.

An Example: Predicting Births of Boys and Girls

Consider the following simple problem (Kahneman & Tversky, 1982):

A certain town is served by two hospitals. In the larger hospital about 45 babies are born each day, and in the smaller hospital about 15 babies are born each day. About 50% of all babies are boys. The exact percentage of baby boys, however, varies from day to day. Sometimes it may be higher than 50%, sometimes lower. For a period of one year, each hospital recorded the days on which more than 60% of the babies born were boys. Which hospital do you think recorded more such days: the larger hospital, the smaller hospital, or did they have about the same number of days?

Although this question may seem simple or even silly, it is actually a carefully designed test of the rationality of the answerer. There is a normative theory of probability that gives a "correct" answer to this problem, but there is also a commonsensical theory that gives a different answer; the intuitive decision maker, limited perceptually and conceptually, uses shortcuts to reason through such problems. Kahneman and Tversky (1972) have thus created a comparison, and it is controlled because answers are produced to a standardized and simple problem. Through such simple but ingenious questions they have demonstrated that people do not reason according to the "rational" model, but rather use a set of informal rules or *heuristics* to make such judgments.

The commonsensical theory says that the two hospitals are doing the same thing in the same way, and should therefore have the same results.

This reasoning by similarity is called the *representative heuristic*. In fact, the majority of undergraduate students answer this problem by saying "Same" (Kahneman & Tversky, 1972). The laws of probability, however, propose that the small hospital will have more variation in proportion of boy babies because each day is based on a smaller number of babies born. Consider that, if the small hospital has only one birth each day, then half of the time it would have *all* boys born that day, and the other half it would have *all* girls born. As the number of babies born each day gets larger, fewer days will have an extreme proportion of boys or girls born. The proper answer to the question, therefore, is that the smaller hospital will have more days with imbalanced births (regardless of whether it is a preponderance of boys or girls).

An Example: Framing Gains and Losses

Consider a second example of this method, this time contrasting answers to two somewhat different questions. First, imagine the following situation (Tversky & Kahneman, 1981):

Imagine that the U.S. is preparing for the outbreak of an unusual Asian disease, which is expected to kill 600 people. Two alternative programs to combat the disease have been proposed. Assume that the exact scientific estimate of the consequences of the programs are as follows:

(A) If program A is adopted, 200 people will be saved.
(B) If program B is adopted, there is a one-third probability that 600 people will be saved, and two-thirds probability that no people will be saved.

Which of the two programs would you favor?

The above question is different from the previous one about babies born in hospitals because there is no right or wrong answer. It is strictly a matter of preference and what economists call *risk attitude*. Consider your answers, however, when you imagine the same situation with two different alternatives:

(C) If program C is adopted, 400 people will die.
(D) If program D is adopted, there is a one-third probability that nobody will die, and two-thirds probability that 600 people will die.

Once again, this is a question with no right or wrong answer. Preferences on this question, however, are intimately connected with preferences on the preceding question because program A is the same as program C, and program B is program D (again, a controlled comparison)! The difference between them is that in the first version lives may be *saved*, whereas in the second version people may *die*; but the same number of people live or die in both versions. A person who prefers one alternative in the first problem should prefer the corresponding alternative in the second problem. Regardless of personal preferences or risk attitudes, the rational decision maker must at least be *consistent*.

As you may have guessed, or as you may have found when you answered the problems, this is not necessarily the case. Tversky and Kahneman (1981) showed that 72% of people took the sure thing (presented as Program A) in order to save at least some lives, and 78% chose the risky option (presented as program D) to try to avoid having people die. Although these "framing effects" have mostly been demonstrated at an aggregate level using between-subject designs, reversals of choice have been shown in within-subjects designs where the same subjects see both versions of the problem.

The reason for these discrepancies is that people do not evaluate options in absolute terms, but instead think in terms of gains and losses from a reference point. The two versions of the problem subtly shift the reference point: in the lives-saved version, the reference point is that people are already "dead"; but in the lives-lost version no one has yet died. According to prospect theory (Kahneman & Tversky, 1979), gains and losses are evaluated on value functions with different shapes. In effect, three $2 million gains are more pleasurable than one $6 million gain, but one $6 million loss is more painful than three $2 million losses (Thaler, 1985).

CONTROLLED DECISION TASKS

Decision researchers frequently are interested in research questions about features of the decision task, as well as the particular attributes of alternatives. For example, do decision makers make better decisions alone or in groups? What happens when there are time constraints? Are better decisions made when information is presented in tabular or graphical form? Such questions could be addressed by examining naturally occurring variations, but one would encounter considerable difficulty in finding events of the right sort and in separating confounding factors. Decision researchers have found experiments to be a useful way to address such

Table 6.1
Lotteries That Produce Reference Reversals

	P-Question	G-Question
Probability of Winning	35/36	11/36
Amount to Win	$4.00	$36.00
Probability of Losing	1/36	25/36
Amount to Lose	$1.00	$1.50

questions about decision tasks (Payne, 1982, summarizes many task contingencies that affect decision making).

An Example: Preference Reversals in
Bidding Versus Choice

A very interesting line of research began twenty years ago with the discovery of a remarkable phenomenon. Slovic and Lichtenstein (1968) asked people to evaluate hypothetical gambles (see Figure 6.1) as either choices or bids. In the choice procedure, decision makers gave their preferences between two gambles (which would they play once if they could play one and only one?). In the bid procedure, they stated the highest prices they would pay to play each gamble once.

The startling results were that particular pairs of gambles reliably produced inconsistent preferences and bids. For example, people preferred to play the P-gamble (called a P-gamble because the probability of winning is high) in Figure 6.1 rather than the G-gamble (called a G-gamble because the gain is high) when given a choice, yet their bids for the G-gamble were consistently higher than for the P-gamble. It is as if they preferred less money to more!

Once this phenomenon came to light, research questions emerged rapidly: (1) Is this a reliable phenomenon? (2) How can we describe which gambles exhibit this reversal? (3) Is the phenomenon important; does it appear in a variety of natural settings? (4) How can we explain the phenomenon; what theories can be found or created that predict such behavior?

The first two questions were answered rapidly by Lichtenstein and Slovic (1971, 1973). They used many examples of gambles in several studies and showed that the phenomenon was reliable. Furthermore, they established the types of gambles that showed such reversals. Specifically, gambles with high probability of winning small amounts (P-gambles) were preferred over gambles with low probability of winning large amounts (G-gambles); but the gambles offering higher gains attracted higher bids than the gambles offering lower gains.

The third question is often the central criticism of the style of research portrayed here. The research is contrived, artificial, and lacks context and actual consequences. In this case, however, Lichtenstein and Slovic (1973) cleverly recreated their experiments in a special room of the Four Queens Casino in Las Vegas. Gamblers were given opportunities to play with real money and without awareness of the special nature of the situation. The results were identical: Preferences between gambles (choices) were inconsistent with what actual gamblers paid to play the gambles (bids).

But why does this phenomenon occur? It is here that theory-building activity becomes most intensive. Slovic and Lichtenstein (1973) proposed that the phenomenon could be explained as an instance of a more general heuristic: anchoring and adjustment (Tversky & Kahneman, 1974). Specifically, the request for a bid in dollars produces a natural tendency to examine the amount to win (in dollars) and adjust this amount downward for the probability of winning and the risk of loss. The anchoring and adjustment process tends to be conservative—that is, adjustments are insufficient, leaving the final bid too close to the anchor. In this case, it leaves the final bids too close to the amount to win, and thus too high.

The alternative process of stating a relative preference between two gambles does not use anchoring and adjustment. Instead, Payne and Braunstein (1971) suggested that there are a series of simple comparisons both within the individual gambles (if the likelihood of winning is greater than the likelihood of losing, then it's a good gamble), and between gambles (which has the greater amount to win?). The result, however, is that in choosing among gambles such as those in Table 6.1 the attributes of the gambles are used in a different way from the anchoring and adjustment rule used in bidding, resulting in systematic inconsistencies between choices and bids.

Subsequently, the preference reversal phenomenon became a very active research area. Two economists, Grether and Plott (1979), tested 13 explanations for preference reversals in a series of experiments. They found, for example, that clearer and more careful instructions, larger monetary incentives, and conducting the experiments by skeptical economists instead of psychologists did not alter the basic phenomenon. In the end, they reluctantly concluded that the anchoring-and-adjustment explanation was the only one that still fit all the facts, including the new facts they had produced with their studies.

The preference reversal phenomenon has seen a significant increase in research through its 20-year history. New theories have been developed (Goldstein & Einhorn, 1987; Tversky, Slovic, & Kahneman, 1990), and have been explored by both experimentation (Casey, 1990) and process approaches (Schkade & Johnson, 1989). The cycle of discovering phenomena, exploring them, explaining them, testing the explanations, predicting new phenomena based on the theories underlying the explanations, and so forth, is never-ending. Theories are pushed to be more specific, more complete, more general, and to fit more facts.

Controlled Comparisons: A Consumer's Guide

The use of hypothetical stimuli and experimental designs offers both advantages and disadvantages. On the one hand, the carefully controlled materials permit precise tests of hypotheses, such as whether decisions are based on configural use of information. The procedure is highly efficient, because one can create decision situations instead of waiting for them to occur naturally—with all the attendant problems of time, cooperation, reactivity, measurement, multicollinearity, and so forth. On the other hand, the decision task may be rather different from real decision tasks, and only a few decision cues can be factorially manipulated before the study gets complex and unwieldy. We discuss three of these issues in more detail: naturalism, theory development, and discovery.

Naturalism

When research tasks are stripped of everyday content and context, there is no guarantee that the research task is relevant to naturalistic decisions. For example, in the diagnosis of ulcer malignancy from hypothetical written cues, how can we know whether the knowledge and motivation of these decision makers was engaged? What features of real X rays and other symptoms were missing from this artificial task? Did it matter that all the information was presented simultaneously, instead of sequentially (although the radiologists may have used the cues sequentially)? Did it matter that the cases in the study did not match the natural distribution of cases? Studies with hypothetical situations tell us what *can* happen, but not always what *does* happen in natural settings with many uncontrolled factors. Such predictions require additional results from more naturalistic studies, or a strong theory specifying which components of a decision are the same in natural and artificial tasks.

Although the use of controlled tasks often conflicts with the desire to use naturalistic materials and situations, it is often possible to create adequate levels of both control and naturalism. For example, a factorial design of attributes could be presented along with other stimuli having a more natural range and combination of attributes, so that the total set of materials is less strange. Of course, the burden on the decision makers increases, because they are making "filler" judgments, but this is usually a manageable problem for researchers. This burden can be reduced by designs such as fractional factorials that present fewer cue combinations but give up tests of some effects (for example, researchers almost never find interactions among four or more cues). Decision materials could be made to look more realistic, with more attention paid to selection of real-world decision makers and realistic consequences. Usually, this means consulting with some practitioners before finalizing materials that are meant to mimic natural decisions, just as Hoffman, Slovic, and Rorer (1968) did in the study of ulcer malignancy diagnosis—a good procedure in any study.

Theory Development

These highly abstract methods are oriented toward identifying *natural laws*—they look for a few variables that will exhibit simple relationships across many situations and many people. They are used when researchers are interested in establishing one theoretical fact, usually a comparison. For example, people are more likely to take financial risks when they believe they are behind or below a given goal or quota than if they are ahead or on target. Individual differences and situational contingencies are treated as "noise" in order to create simple and controlled tasks. Over time and many research studies, the noise is gradually partitioned into theoretical constructs and variables that can be tested one at a time after the basic phenomena are established. This strategy is most useful when the researcher has a highly structured problem with well-specified research questions or predictions and only a few known variables of interest.

These techniques are like telescopes that are able to reveal the detailed structure of decision and judgment, but have to be focused at the right objects—objects already known to the researcher. For example, the question-answering technique has been very successful at providing lists of errors and biases that strain normative theory. It has been less effective however, at identifying the sources of frames and heuristics in the cognitive processes underlying decision making. How do people decide what is a gain or a loss, and what frames other than gains and losses matter in formulating a decision problem? How do we know which heuristics exist? Where do heuristics come from, and do decision makers have to choose among them?

Discovery

Researchers interested in discovering new phenomena and processes, uncovering interesting variables and situations, or creating experiments that interweave all the features of a situation to explain and predict specific behavior typically adopt a different style of research. The self-report and case methods discussed in Chapter 3 are better suited to dealing with naturalistic phenomena and discovery. Under some circumstances, the methods presented in Chapter 4 and Chapter 5 can also lead to surprises and discoveries. There is no substitute, however, for a keen observer with an open mind, an inquiring attitude, and a willingness to use whatever methods best fit the topics and questions of interest.

SKILL BUILDING

1. Think about whether groups make better decisions than do individuals. Let's take as an example a hiring situation. Should potential job candidates be evaluated by one person or by a panel? The only justification for a more time-consuming process is some enhancement of quality.

   (a) What is meant by a "better" decision? Define for yourself what it means in this situation (e.g., performance against criteria, avoidance of bias, conformity to normative models, consideration of more relevant factors). If you were dealing with a real hiring situation, how would you find out what "better" means?

   (b) Design a study in which hypothetical job applicants are evaluated by individuals or groups. What kinds of stimuli would be used, and how would they be selected? How big a group would you use? What decisions or judgmental responses would be requested? How would you know if groups were better than individuals?

   (c) How could you make the evaluation of hypothetical job applicants as realistic, natural, and involving as possible? How would you design stimuli, instructions, rewards, and select decision makers in order to enhance ecological validity?

(d) What confounds have been controlled, and which, if any, are still troublesome? In what ways has this design permitted stronger comparisons than in a study of existing hiring decisions, and in what ways does it fall short?

2. Design an experiment to see whether the differences between gains and losses demonstrated with small bets (usually in the range of $1 to $100) would also occur with large bets (personnel or business situations in which large sums of money are at stake).

(a) It is relatively easy to design a study by taking the materials of previous research and multiplying all amounts by 100. Make sure, however, that you create a comparison between small and large amounts, as well as between bids and choices.

(b) How would you make this study as realistic and involving as possible?

7

Problems in Applications

No matter how well-trained in research methodology one is, the actual use of research methods takes place in a broader context. This is particularly important if the research utilizes participants who have not acquiesced to the "scientific culture" (e.g., college students who know they have to take part in research), or takes researchers into a field setting outside of their own "turf." The purpose of this chapter is to raise some practical and political issues that determine whether research can be carried out, and the resultant quality and usefulness of the research products.

In this chapter, we will discuss four problems that frequently emerge in decision research: access and cooperation, evaluation apprehension, the use and misuse of research results, and ethics.

ACCESS AND COOPERATION

Research can be carried out on one's own turf, that is, where the researcher has the authority and the legitimacy to do the job, or on other people's turf, where the researcher is an intruder who is probably interfering with the legitimate work and the informal arrangements of others. Problems with access and cooperation are obviously much more serious outside one's own turf. The researcher has to be sensitive to the stakeholders and their agendas, and to the acceptable means for soliciting or coercing cooperation.

Some of our research habits and mental frameworks emerged when research was carried out with college student "subjects" who were "run" through experiments, using the metaphor of research with laboratory rats. We are better served by the metaphor of *collaboration:* research participants are colleagues or experts in their own right who share their insights with the researcher(s) and permit access to settings, records, and their own thoughts and behaviors.

Probably the best advice is to put oneself in the role of each type of stakeholder in the setting: How can you help them or harm them? For example, will your research be seen as an evaluation of decision making,

Table 7.1

Letter to Potential Research Participants

Dear Sir or Madam:

How do you make decisions? Do you plan and calculate, use intuition, or just react? Scientists and policy makers need a better understanding of how people make complex real decisions such as taxpaying.

As Director of the M.I.T. Taxpayer Decision Making Research Project, which is funded by the National Science Foundation, I invite you to help us by participating in a study of how taxpayers make decisions about reporting and paying their personal taxes. Here are some good reasons why you should participate:

- You can contribute to the scientific study of decision making.
- Your opinions will be heard. You can have a real impact on tax policy.
- We need YOU so that the results will correctly represent all taxpayers.
- We will pay you $100 or donate $100 to the charity of your choice.
- You will have little extra to do—you do your taxes in the usual way.
- Whatever you tell us is strictly confidential. The steps we arc taking to insure your privacy are described on the next page.

We welcome your interest in this research no matter whether you feel that the personal tax laws are fair or unfair, if you work hard at following the full "letter of the law" or if you try to reduce your taxes in every possible way.

If you are interested in participating in the research, then fill in the enclosed REPLY FORM and send it to me in the next few days. We will contact you to explain the rest of the study. If someone else in your household is responsible for personal taxes, then please give them this material.

Thank you for your cooperation. Please call me or write to me if you have any questions or comments.

Sincerely yours,
John S. Carroll

---

in which case those afraid of "flunking the test" may withhold cooperation or even undermine the research? Cooperation may be perceived as a waste of time if you emphasize how little you know about the substance of their decision making! Will participants perceive you to be working for a senior manager, reporting back inefficiencies or discontent?

As an example of practical considerations in gaining cooperation, Table 7.1 shows an actual letter sent from one of the authors of this book to potential research participants. The letter requested voluntary cooperation in a project studying taxpayer decision making (Carroll, in press), clearly a very sensitive and personal topic. The letter attempted to bring up positive reasons for taking part in the study, and to alleviate concerns about negative outcomes of participation. Copies of this letter were sent to a stratified random sample of taxpayers in the Boston area, approximately 15% of whom signed and returned the consent form as volunteers. Although this response rate is low compared to simple surveys, it is high for soliciting volunteers to take part in a lengthy and sensitive project potentially exposing them to legal risks (for example, a majority admitted to cheating on their taxes in the past three years).

Some decision research methods demand high levels of cooperation and time on the part of the decision maker. Often, when faced with research that busy experts do not want, they will use time demands as a convenient excuse for not participating. In these circumstances, the best that the researcher can do is to minimize the time demands, and to make clear to the decision makers *why* their investment of time is worthwhile. In general, variations of a method can be constructed to allow decision research under time pressure (such as the fractional factorial design mentioned in Chapter 6). Adapting these methods takes creativity and understanding, but the potential benefits make it worth the effort.

EVALUATION APPREHENSION

In addition to being time-consuming, decision research sometimes can be threatening. There are two major reasons for this: First, decision makers who are insecure about their performance will be concerned that they are being evaluated and may be found wanting. Second, the decision rules that decision makers actually use may be very different from those that they say they use. We will provide some examples of both these issues and offer some suggestions for how to deal with them.

Evaluating and Replacing Decision Makers

In many domains, decision making is a difficult task because the situation is very complex and inherently uncertain; decision makers such as stock analysts, personnel officers, or loan officers will have limited ability to predict outcomes. For example, parole decision makers' predictions of post-release outcomes in actual cases were hardly better than guesswork; even the best predictive models had limited value, although they outperformed the experts (Carroll, Wiener, Coates, Galegher, & Alibrio, 1982).

Clearly, the analyst who finds that the decision maker's performance is poor in some absolute sense faces a problem. By itself, the fact that experts cannot predict particularly well should not be overly disturbing to the expert: The analyst can point out that the task itself is quite difficult, and that prediction in a number of other tasks where experts are employed is difficult. The optimistic outcome would be a more modest decision maker. Realistically, though, the result runs counter to the experts' intuitions, training, and reputation: "That isn't really what we do . . ." is a surprisingly common attempt to disregard the research.

A more serious problem occurs when a model is better than the decision maker, and therefore capable of replacing the experts. The literature provides many examples of potentially embarrassing evaluations of experts, based on the surprisingly good performance of simple linear regression models (Dawes, 1974; Dawes, Faust, & Meehl, 1989). The experts can be surprisingly confident of their abilities, and reject the researcher's conclusions. Discussing the results requires some sensitivity and a knowledge of the political environment in which the experts operate. There seem to be two strategies, however, which may minimize the conflict between research results and the experts' role.

First, the researcher can suggest that a model might work in partnership with the experts, providing an aid rather than a replacement. In the case of the parole board, a guideline system (based on prior work for the U.S. Parole Commission by Gottfredson, Wilkins, & Hoffman, 1978) was created that provided presumptive decisions based on the model but permitted the experts to override the model in specific cases, and to update the rules within the model through a policy-making process. Similarly, Batterymarch (the financial analysis firm discussed in Chapter 2) uses mathematical models to screen securities and pick stocks from this pre-screened list, but the rules in the model are created and tested by their expert securities analysts. The computer only implements what people have created, and provides a tool for that creativity. Combining models and experts is often politically viable because experts are not replaced but, rather, are aided by the models. If there is sufficient valid information in the environment that is known to the experts, but not in the model, then the combination can exceed the model alone (Blattberg & Hosh, in press; Johnson, 1988).

A second strategy is to emphasize that an expert's job often involves more than simply prediction. A financial analyst or a physician, for example, must also maintain good relations with clients. Thus, a model cannot fully replace such an expert, but must be thought of as an aid or an assistant to the decision maker. The analyst can suggest that the expert is now free to concentrate on other parts of the job. In any case, a sensitivity to these potential problems may make the difference between research that itself makes a difference and research that is ignored.

Making Decision Rules Explicit

The criteria used for making important decisions often are controversial. They may reflect the values of the decision maker, but not necessarily those of a wider set of political constituents. Decision research can uncover skeletons and cut through the security of ambiguity. For example, consider a study of how physicians select residents and interns at a well-known teaching hospital (Johnson, 1988). The study, conducted by the second author of this book, examined a large number of decisions and built regression models predicting the ratings that each of the 12 members of the admissions committee would give for the applicants. The models provided an unexpected and controversial result: Two of the physicians on the committee seemed to be markedly sexist because they rated female applicants significantly lower than similar male applicants.

The researcher, who was perhaps more naive and idealistic at the time, simply reported the facts at a research presentation without revealing the identity of the physicians. To the hospital's credit, they reacted in a positive and constructive manner: The study had also found that a small committee would save effort, yet be just as good at selecting interns; next year's smaller committee simply excluded the two offending judges. These results confirmed the suspicions of other committee members, and the identity of the sexist physicians was easily surmised.

Had the doctors been less enlightened, however, or the offending doctors in more powerful positions, the result might have been quite different. The researcher might have been told that he was wrong, and banned from any further access to this hospital. Furthermore, he might have lost the opportunity to have a beneficial impact upon the decision-making process. Even more dramatically, the researcher might have been sued for slander, defamation of character, or whatever a clever attorney and an angry physician could have dreamed up.

THE USE AND MISUSE OF RESEARCH

There is no guarantee that data collected will be properly interpreted, or that research conducted will be used in a way that is consistent with the data and the interpretations of the researcher. Research may be used by organizations in much the same way as consultants are used: If the results agree with what was believed, then actions will be implemented and supported with arguments based on the research; on the other hand, if the results are not in agreement with prior beliefs, then the research report may end up buried in file drawers and ignored.

In a very interesting study, Lord, Ross, and Lepper (1979) showed that the interpretation of research evidence strongly depends on the prior beliefs of the audience. When subjects favoring one side of an issue were presented with two research studies (one with results supporting their side, and the other with results opposing their side) they tended to believe the supportive results and to criticize the methodology of the study opposing their views. After reading both studies, the participants' beliefs in their prior views actually became stronger. This occurred for supporters of both sides of the issue, and occurred regardless of whether it was a lab study or a field study that supported their side. The conclusion is clear: Research cannot be viewed as neutral, and the interpretation of research cannot be counted on to remain neutral or objective.

As a second example of this process, consider the use of social science research by the courts. Beginning with *Brown v. Board of Education*, the courts have increasingly included research results in support of their opinions. They have tended to interpret the research to suit their own needs, however, and not to create an objective portrayal of *scientific knowledge*. For example, in the 1970s the United States Supreme Court decided a series of cases about the permissible number of jurors for various types of cases. As Grofman and Scarrow (1980) observe,

> The empirical studies that the Court (or at least Justice Blackmun) relied upon in *Ballew* to declare *five*-member juries unconstitutional were in fact studies which compared *six*-member juries and *12*-member juries . . . For Justice Blackmun to then come out in opposition to five-member juries and to reaffirm his support for six-member juries seems, to put it mildly, to have been disingenuous. (p. 121)

Thus, although the Supreme Court's decisions appear to be based on social science research, they are more likely to represent a marshalling of arguments by the court for opinions they have made on other grounds.

Researchers themselves interpret results in ways that confirm their prior beliefs, and choose to study topics in ways that reflect implicit assumptions. For example, decades of research on race differences primarily investigated the relationship between personal characteristics of whites and blacks and various achievements, but did not study the characteristics of the environments in which whites and blacks lived. As a result, the research could only conclude that whites and blacks were different because of personal characteristics (or find no difference) but could say nothing about environmental causes of these differences (Caplan & Nelson, 1973). Similarly, if we choose to study decisions as the product of individual values and preferences, we have made some implicit assumptions that cannot be tested without collecting a very different kind of data.

ETHICS

A researcher may turn up information that would harm someone if it were revealed. Decision makers could lose their jobs if the low quality of their decisions was revealed; sexist and racist behaviors could come to light that organizations have been trying to keep secret or to change in gradual ways. Information could be revealed that would be seen as an invasion of privacy, or as violating pledges of confidentiality extended to research participants. These are not only practical issues; they are also ethical and legal issues.

Earlier in this chapter we discussed a situation in which a researcher discovered that some decision makers were sexist (in violation of the law). Are researchers required to turn in their information? If a researcher has made an agreement with an organization and individual participants that confidentiality will be preserved—meaning that the identities of the participants will not be revealed and cannot be attached to the results—is the researcher obligated *not* to present the data in a way that reveals, for example, sexism? What if the researcher is being paid by the organization, or works for it, or was hired by someone who turns out to be the offending decision maker, or has a strong interest in continuing to do research at the same site for many years?

These situations raise a set of overlapping and inconsistent obligations—to the research participants, to personal relationships, to the organization that paid for the research, to science, to professional societies, to society in general, to the law, to oneself, and to morality or religion. There are no hard and fast rules for resolving these conflicts. Professional organizations have ethical principles to help guide their members, but these can be vague or inconsistent as well. It is not the principles, but rather their application to specific cases that is problematic.

SOME ADVICE

Probably the best advice that can be offered is to think through the possible conflicts and work out the obligations as explicitly as possible *before* doing the research. Who will control publication of the results? What if one turns up an incompetent decision maker? Is it the researcher's job to blow the whistle on an incompetent, or only if something illegal or harmful is going on?

A second piece of advice is to involve relevant others in developing a political and ethical analysis of a project. Researchers are too close to the problem and have natural biases about their own research; they need their perceptions checked and broadened by colleagues and those affected by the research. For example, Rosenbaum et al. (1979) observed shoppers in retail stores, and some of the shoppers actually shoplifted. The legal and ethical dilemmas were eased greatly by prior discussions with store security personnel, who instructed the research team not to interfere with shoplifters. They explained that it was their job to intervene, and that the researchers would open themselves and the store to legal action. Furthermore, the research would contribute most by providing information about shoplifting and theories of decision making, not by apprehending a few shoplifters.

Finally, it may be helpful to structure the collective understanding about the project in the form of a written document. Although contracts are a typical form of agreement for consulting arrangements, research projects are usually arranged verbally. Unfortunately, there remains possibilities for later misinterpretation, attempts to apply pressure, and changes brought about by movement of key personnel. A reasonable idea is to embody the main points of the agreement in a letter, copies of which are kept by key parties. This would include statements about the role of the researcher, control of data collection, ownership of the data, rights of publication, and so forth.

Thus, the practical, political, and ethical considerations we have raised in this chapter are factors all researchers confront at some time in their projects. Some learn from painful experience; some are lucky and do not get burned. The best advice is to plan and think ahead, and to discuss the potential issues with experienced researchers and representatives of the various constituencies that one is studying, working with, and working for.

SKILL BUILDING

1. Imagine someone was beginning a project on personnel decisions (hiring, promotions) made in the organization in which you work or study.
   (a) What could they found out that could help or hurt people in the organization? Could anything affect you?
   (b) Would you be willing to cooperate in the research? Why or why not? Under what circumstances would you be more or less willing to cooperate?
2. Imagine that you plan to study how law firms decide to promote associates to partners. Your plan is to involve several firms in two studies: (1) a retrospective analysis of past decisions based on existing records, and (2) an experiment in which hypothetical associates with manipulated characteristics are "evaluated" for partnership by the partners themselves. Answer the following questions:
   (a) Who are the constituencies that should be consulted and who must cooperate in order for you to gain access? What would these groups want from you and what would they be concerned about? How would you set up an agreement about the project?
   (b) How might the results of this research be of interest to the various constituencies? What practical applications might emerge? Are there ways in which the research could be misinterpreted or misused? Why might this happen, and how could it be avoided?
   (c) Are there any ethical issues? If so, what could be done to deal with them or head them off?
3. What do you think should be the role of decision research in society? How do you think the conflicting claims of the law, professional groups, science, ethics, personal career, and others should be evaluated?

8

Summary and Future Directions

Throughout this book, we have tried to bring out the advantages and disadvantages of a variety of decision research methods, and ways to cope with or minimize the disadvantages. We begin our summary with a simultaneous comparison of all the major methods. We hope this will reemphasize the important considerations, and our best guesses about the costs and benefits involved. Afterwards, we make a plea for using a *combination* of methods instead of choosing among them. Finally, we consider what the futures holds for decision-making research.

EVALUATING DECISION RESEARCH METHODS

In Chapter 1, we presented six criteria for the benefits and costs of decision research:

1. *Discovery*—having the power to uncover new phenomena, surprise the researcher, and lead to creative insights.
2. *Understanding*—providing a cause-and-effect analysis that uncovers the mechanisms or processes by which decisions are made.
3. *Prediction*—having logical or mathematical rules that predict the judgments and decisions that will be made. These rules may predict without capturing the actual decision processes.
4. *Prescriptive Control*—providing opportunities and techniques for changing the decision process, as in prescribing decision rules or testing potential manipulations.
5. *Confound Control*—creating controlled decision situations so as to rule out other explanations of the results (known as *confounds*).
6. *Ease of Use*—taking less time and resources for the same progress toward the other goals.

Table 8.1 summarizes our evaluations of the major classes of methods: self-report; case; alternative-focused weighted-additive models; attribute-focused weighted-additive models; verbal protocols; search;

Table 8.1
Evaluation of Decision Research Methods

Method	Discovery	Understanding	Prediction	Prescriptive Control	Confound Control	Ease of Use
Self-Report	+	+				++
Case	+	++	Local	Local		
Alternative		+	++	+	+	+
Attribute			+	++	+	
Protocols	+	++				
Search		++				
Q/A		+			+	+
Experiments		++	+	++	++	
Lab/Field	Field	?	Field	?	Lab	Lab

question-answering; and experiments. In addition, because many of these methods can be used with varying levels of realism, the table includes a contrast between using these methods in the field (or with real situations) against using them in the laboratory (or with hypothetical situations).

There is a critical caveat associated with this table: No method can really be scored in a simple way on these criteria. Any research method can be used well or poorly, intensively or casually, creatively or by rote, and applied in different ways to different research situations. The evaluations in the table are a starting point for thoughtful consideration, not a decision rule for choosing a research method!

Discovery

Exploration requires unstructured techniques, although there may be a lot of "technique" and experienced know-how underlying the apparent lack of structure. Self-report methods, case studies, and verbal protocols are less structured. They permit situations to speak for themselves, and therefore have a better chance of finding out information that was unanticipated or perhaps not part of the original studies at all. The other methods are more structured, rigorous, more apparently "scientific," but create some rigidity along with the structure.

Understanding

There is a lot of debate over what is meant by "understanding" or what sort of models are desirable in the study of decision making. What most behavioral decision theorists mean by understanding is a model that captures intervening processes, exemplified by process-tracing techniques such as verbal protocols and search methods. Other reference traditions, however, look for detailed understanding through self-reports, intensive case studies, and carefully designed experiments.

Prediction

Weighted-additive models, particularly alternative-focused techniques, are designed to predict decisions with high accuracy. Sometimes this accuracy is embarrassing to the human experts who are the subjects of the research. Experiments also provide prediction, but tend to make relative predictions (how conditions will differ) rather than absolute predictions. Case studies can provide good prediction for the case at hand, but tend to be weak at generalizing to other instances. This is why case studies are evaluated as good for "local" predictions.

Prescriptive Control

Weighted-additive models also are useful for aiding or replacing decision makers. Attribute-focused techniques are particularly well-designed to help decision makers use a normative model such as utility theory or Bayesian statistics. Experiments offer precise comparisons between new and old ways of deciding. Case studies once again may permit strong prescriptions for specific cases, but their usefulness may drop rapidly unless representative cases have been studied.

Confound Control

Experiments have the strongest controls against extraneous factors. Experiments can only look at a few things at a time, however, because they are so busy controlling everything. Weighted-additive models are developed using methods that have strong controls, although more naturalistic versions of these methods begin to give up much of this control.

Ease of Use

Self-reports are usually easy to get. This is typically the way research begins, and often the way it ends. Question-answering is a little more difficult because the questions must be carefully designed. Some types of experiments and case studies are relatively easy to do, but others are quite laborious. Weighted-additive models tend to be moderately easy to create, whereas process-tracing techniques are of moderate to high difficulty. Naturally, these evaluations depend greatly on the specifics of the studies.

Field/Real Versus Lab/Hypothetical

There are weighted-additive models developed using hypothetical decision situations, and ones based upon actual decisions by actual decision makers. The real situations are likely to be higher in the criteria of discovery, prediction, and prescriptive control, but lower on confound control and ease of use. It is not clear how to evaluate understanding in any simple way.

Similarly, protocols, search methods, and experiments can be conducted with hypothetical situations in laboratories, or with real situations in field settings. The same sorts of trade-offs are likely to occur. Contrast, for example, collecting verbal protocols from managers presented with an in-basket exercise of hypothetical situations, with protocols from managers actually doing their jobs (both are used by Isenberg, in press).

The hypothetical situations offer the advantages of ease of use (they take less time and can be scheduled at the researcher's convenience), confound control (the in-basket can be carefully designed and is given to everyone in controlled settings), and some possibility for understanding features that could be carefully built into the situations (for example, testing differences between scenarios).

The in vivo collection of protocols is more difficult and unpredictable. Yet, for the same reasons, it offers more opportunities for discovery, is likely to be a better predictor of what managers really do, and may enhance understanding of the broader view of managerial decision making.

COMBINING METHODS

The above analysis seems to suggest that the researcher is caught in a dilemma: no matter what method is chosen, there are some weaknesses that must be endured (McGrath, 1982). We acknowledge that *all* the criteria cannot be fully addressed in a single study. Researchers must choose, depending on their goals for the study and assessment of situations and their own skills. The field of decision research, however, permits a kind of teamwork among separate researchers. If different studies utilizing different methods are conducted in ways that overlap their research questions, then the combined evidence of many studies can overcome their individual weaknesses.

This leads to the paradoxical statement that methods need not be chosen for use because they are accepted, proven, or otherwise successful. From the viewpoint of the individual researcher, such success is a good reason for sticking with the "tried and true." But from the broader viewpoint of the field of decision research, the accepted method may contain a flaw that will only be revealed when someone uses a different method.

There is a second answer to achieving all the goals of research, namely, to use multiple methods in the same study or project. For example, although a single case study has many weaknesses for generalizing beyond the case, a few well-chosen cases permit much stronger comparisons and greatly increase our level of understanding, prediction, and potential for control. This is a simple mix of case methods with controlled comparisons.

Similarly, weighted-additive models can be mixed with process-tracing techniques. The simplest way is to collect verbal protocols from a subset of the subjects or a subset of the decisions from which the weighted-additive models are derived. This gives an opportunity to look at decision processes in more depth and discover new insights, while preserving the strengths of the weighted-additive models. For example, Johnson and Schkade (1989) show that different strategies, revealed by verbal protocols and search methods, help predict differences in the amount of bias demonstrated in utility assessment.

Protocol and search methods can be combined with controlled comparisons of decision situations, and self-report and case methods can be introduced to examine the broader context in which these decisions occur. In short, all combinations are possible, limited only by the creativity of the researcher and the resources available.

There is one criterion that cannot be met if methods are to be combined: ease of use. Studies with such methodological innovations will be more complex and time-consuming; they will require more cooperation from research participants and more skill on the part of the researchers. It is not surprising that researchers tend to specialize in some familiar methods, to interact with other researchers who use the same methods, and to believe increasingly that their preferred methods are best. Researchers who expand their range of skills or collaborate with other researchers who specialize in different methods, however, should reap substantial benefits and lead the field of decision research into the future.

THE FUTURE OF DECISION RESEARCH

The methods of decision research that we have presented in this book include techniques that have been used for centuries, and some that are only a few years old. Progress in the study of decision making has accelerated tremendously in the last 20 years, and a book about decision research methods 10 years from now will most likely look quite different from this one.

Part of the rapid pace of change is due to technological advances. Herbert Simon has remarked that his studies of problem solving depended on the invention of the tape recorder, so that verbal protocols could be collected and studied in detail. Process-tracing methods—the most recent addition to the portfolio of decision research techniques—depend upon tape recorders, chronometers, eye-movement apparatus, and computers with various capabilities for displaying and recording information. Even theory development has begun to use the metaphor of the computer and to express theories as computer programs.

In this closing section of the book, we look ahead to the future of decision making and decision-making research. We speculate about two different aspects of the impact of technology: first, how the methods and theories of decision research will change as new technologies become available, and second, how decision making itself will change as decision makers utilize these new technologies. We outline some areas worth watching, and examine some of the opportunities that will be presented by the development of new technologies in other disciplines.

Artificial Intelligence

The field of artificial intelligence attempts to address some issues that are related closely to decision research. In expert system development, the goal is to build a computer representation that will make judgments and decisions much like those of experts. One example would be the MYCIN system (Shortliffe & Buchanan, 1984), which diagnoses bacteriological infections and selects appropriate antibiotic therapies.

Most expert systems employ a set of if-then rules, each of which pecify that if a certain condition is true, then a certain action is per-ormed. In MYCIN, the system may ask about the age and the symptoms f the patient and (depending upon the results) ask about data from arious clinical tests. This is in sharp contrast to regression models that onsider the same kind of information for each case, and more like the gical strategies and heuristics that were discussed in Chapter 5.

Expert systems are built through interactions with decision makers, sking them how they solve problems. This process, which is sometimes alled *knowledge extraction*, is time-consuming and laborious. Yet, while seems to have something in common with the process-tracing tech- iques discussed in Chapter 5, knowledge extraction is seldom done on a ormal basis. It has more of the character of an interview—such as those iscussed in Chapter 3—in which the researcher constructs a system, talks bout it with the decision maker, and then modifies the system.

Another type of artificial intelligence system, rule-induction algo- thms, simply looks at a set of decisions made by the decision maker and uilds a model that would make similar decisions, without claiming that e model represents the details of the underlying cognitive process. For xample, Currim, Meyer, and Le (1988) developed a rule-induction algo- thm to predict which apartments would be acceptable to a potential nter; the model made predictions comparable in quality to those made y one form of weighted-additive model, conjoint analysis.

utomated Decision Analysis

Decision research frequently has been criticized for emphasizing ra- onal—or at least analytical and systematic—processes at the expense of tuition and holistic thinking. Our laboratory tasks seem to force decision akers to look at information in analytical and even quantitative ways. nterestingly, as computer software is developed to aid decision making, e software also emphasizes the analytical side of decision making. The et result is that these decision aids make the world more like the boratory that scientists have created in their own image.

Computerized decision aids are proliferating at a rapid rate. It is ossible now for consumers to shop by using a dial-up system to specify decision rule, and to have that rule screen all the possible alternatives. omp-U-Store, for example, allows a consumer to screen all possible CRs and to list only those that meet certain criteria, such as having ow-motion capabilities, wireless remote controls, and a price of less an $300.

Similarly, software is now available that allows the decision maker to specify a decision rule on a personal computer, and will identify which of a set of options is best. MASS, developed at the Wharton School of Business, allows prospective MBAs to evaluate cities as places to live and work. General-purpose decision aids such as Lightyear and Texas Instruments' Arborist encourage people to analyze alternatives, outcomes, and values systematically.

This new technology makes the standard agenda of decision research more important than ever. The simple decision problems that are so easy to use in laboratory experiments—and criticized as unrelated to real decision making (Konecni & Ebbesen, 1979)—now look quite similar to what the new technologies require of real decision makers. Asking a decision maker to specify a choice rule, or to put a weight on the air quality of cities, is just what researchers have done for years in laboratory settings. Thus, laboratory research may have a surprising amount of relevance to the development of such decision-support systems.

New Data Opportunities

An even more exciting consequence of the new technologies is that they provide unique opportunities for gathering data for decision research. Computer mail, for example, offers a rich data base for understanding group and organizational decision making. We can track the communication of real decision makers simply by recording the flow and contents of mail.

We can illustrate this possibility by contrasting two governmental scandals. Questions about who made what kind of decisions and when these decisions were made were central to both the Watergate and the Iran-Contra investigations. In Watergate, the key to understanding culpability may have been erased in an 18-minute gap on an audiotape. In contrast, during the Iran-Contra affair, computer mail provided a detailed trace of the communication among the participants. This record, to the chagrin of those involved, was quite complete and evaded their attempt to delete crucial items. Although copies of mail were erased, backup copies were easily obtained from standard archives of the computer system. The possibility that computer archives will be part of presidential libraries does not seem farfetched.

In this manner, individual decision makers can be studied by observing their information acquisitions as they access information provided by computers. Automated recording of the information examined provides a powerful, passive, and unobtrusive means of gathering data on decision processes. Such data traps will soon allow the kind of analysis formerly done with information display boards and eye-movement machines to be done in much more realistic settings. Of course, difficult ethical issues regarding privacy are raised at the same time.

Onward and Upward

There is substantial cause for optimism and excitement about the future of decision research. The field has seen explosive growth in the last 10 to 20 years as powerful tools have been developed for studying and aiding decision making. We believe that behavioral decision research, as a field, can make substantial contributions to improving decision making, ranging from small and seemingly unimportant decisions such as which brand of cereal to buy to more immediately important ones such as medical diagnoses, responses in negotiations, or choices among alternative public policies. Our optimism is based, in part, on what has been done in a relatively short period of time. It is also based, however, on the prospects for new developments inspired by new information technologies. Although we have tried to present the state of the art in this book, we also hope we have inspired readers to help make this book obsolete as quickly as possible.

References

belson, R. P., & Levi, A. (1985). Decision making and decision theory. In G. Lindzay & E. Aronson (Eds.), *The handbook of social psychology, 3rd Ed.* New York: Random House.

jzen, I., & Fishbein, M. (1975). *Belief, attitude, intention, and behavior: An introduction to theory and research.* Reading, MA: Addison-Wesley.

llison, G. T. (1971). *The essence of decision: Explaining the Cuban missile crisis.* Boston: Little, Brown.

llport, G. (1937). *Personality: A psychological interpretation.* New York: Henry Holt.

nderson, J. R. (1985). *Cognitive psychology and its implications (2nd ed.).* San Francisco: W. H. Freeman.

nderson, N. H. (1981). *Foundations of information integration theory.* New York: Academic Press.

rgote, L., Seabright, M. A., & Dyer, L. (1986). Individual versus group use of base-rate and individuating information. *Organizational Behavior and Human Decision Processes, 38,* 65-75.

rgyris, C. (1976). Leadership, learning, and changing the status quo. *Organizational Dynamics,* Winter, 29-43.

rgyris, C., & Schon, D. (1974). *Theory in practice: Increasing professional effectiveness.* San Francisco: Jossey-Bass.

rkes, H. R., & Hammond, K. (Eds.). (1986). *Judgment and decision making: An interdisciplinary reader.* Cambridge: Cambridge University.

akwin, H. (1945). Pseudodoxia pediatrica. *New England Journal of Medicine, 232,* 691-697.

azerman, M. H. (1986). *Judgment in managerial decision making.* New York: John Wiley.

azerman, M. H., Giuliano, T., & Appelman, A. (1984). Escalation in individual and group decision making. *Organizational Behavior and Human Performance, 33,* 141-152.

azerman, M. H., Mannix, E., Sondak, H., & Thompson, L. (1990). Negotiator behavior and decision processes in dyads, groups, and markets. In J. S. Carroll (Ed.), *Applied social psychology and organizational settings.* Hillsdale, NJ: Lawrence Erlbaum.

each, L. R., & Mitchell, T. R. (1978). A contingency model for the selection of decision strategies. *Academy of Management Review, 3,* 439-449.

eihal, G., & Charkravarti, D. (1982). Information presentation format and learning goals as determinants of consumers' memory retrieval and choice processes. *Journal of Consumer Research, 8,* 431-441.

ennett, T., & Wright, R. (1984). *Burglars on burglary.* Brookfield, VT: Gower.

ettman, J. R. (1979). *An information processing theory of consumer choice.* Reading, MA: Addison-Wesley.

ettman, J. R., & Park, C. W. (1980). Effects of prior knowledge, exposure, and phase of the choice processes on consumer decision processes: A protocol analysis. *Journal of Consumer Research, 7,* 234-248.

attberg, R. C., & Hoch, S. J. (in press). Database models and managerial intuition: 50% database + 50% manager. *Management Science.*

125

Blumstein, A. (1983). Models for structuring taxpayer compliance. In P. Sawicki (Ed *Income tax compliance: A report of the ABA section of taxation, invitational conferen on income tax compliance*. Washington, DC: American Bar Association.

Bradburn, N. M., Rips, L. J., & Shevell, S. K. (1987). Answering autobiographic questions: The impact of memory and inference on surveys. *Science, 236*, 157-161.

Brunswik, E. (1955). Representative design and probabilistic theory in a functional ps chology. *Psychological Review, 62*(3), 193-217.

Burton, S., & Blair, E. (1986). *Proceedings of the American Statistical Association.*

Campbell, D. T. (1979). "Degrees of freedom" and the case study. In T. D. Cook & C. Reichardt (Eds.), *Qualitative and quantitative methods in evaluation research.* Beve: Hills, CA: Sage.

Caplan, N., & Nelson, S. (1973). On being useful: The nature and consequences psychological research on social problems. *American Psychologist, 28*, 199-211.

Carlsmith, J. M., Ellsworth, P., & Aronson, E. (1978). *Methods of research in soc psychology.* Reading, MA: Addison-Wesley.

Carroll, J. S. (in press). Taxation: Compliance with personal income tax laws. In D. Kagehiro & W. S. Laufer (Eds.), *Handbook of psychology and law.* New York: Spring

Carroll, J. S., Wiener, R., Coates, D., Galegher, J., & Alibrio, J. J. (1982). Evaluati diagnosis, and prediction in parole decision making. *Law and Society Review, .* 199-228.

Casey, J. T. (1990). Reversal of the preference reversal phenomenon. *Organizatior Behavior and Human Decision Processes.*

Cattin, P., & Wittick, D. R. (1982). Commercial use of conjoint analysis: A survey. *Jourr of Marketing, 46*, 44-53.

Clarkson, G. P. E. (1962). *Portfolio selection—a simulation of trust investment.* Englewo Cliffs, NJ: Prentice-Hall.

Cochran, W. G., & Cox, G. M. (1957). *Experimental designs* (2nd Ed.). New York: Jc Wiley.

Connolly, T. (1982). On taking action seriously: Cognitive fixation in behavioral decisi theory. In G. R. Ungson & D. N. Braunstein (Eds.), *Decision making: An interdiscip nary inquiry.* Boston: Kent.

Cook, R. L., & Stewart, T. R. (1975). A comparison of seven methods for obtaini subjective descriptions of judgmental policy. *Organizational Behavior and Hum Performance, 13*, 31-45.

Corbin, R. (1980). Decisions that might not get made. In T. S. Wallsten (Ed.), *Cognit processes in choice and decision behavior* (pp. 47-68). Hillsdale, NJ: Lawrer Erlbaum.

Currim, I., Meyer, R., & Le, N. (1987). A concept learning system for the inference production models of consumer choice. In W. Henry, M. Meansco, & C. Takada (Ed *New product development and testing.* Lexington, MA: Lexington.

Cyert, R. M., & March, J. G. (1963). *A behavioral theory of the firm.* Englewood Clii NJ: Prentice-Hall.

Daft, R. L. (1984). Antecedents of significant and not-so-significant organizational search. In T. S. Bateman & G. R. Ferris (Eds.), *Method and analysis in organizatio research.* Reston, VA: Reston Publishing.

Davis, J. H. (1973). Group decision and social interaction: A theory of social decis schemes. *Psychological Review, 80*, 97-125.

Dawes, R. M. (1971). A case study of graduate admissions: Application of three princip of human decision making. *American Psychologist, 26*, 180-188.

Dawes, R. M. (1979). The robust beauty of improper linear models in decision making. *American Psychologist, 34*, 571-582.

Dawes, R. (1988). *Rational choice in an uncertain world.* New York: Harcourt Brace Jovanovich.

Dawes, R., & Corrigan, B. (1974). Linear models in decision making. *Psychological Bulletin, 81*, 95-106.

Dawes, R., Faust, D., & Meehl, P. E. (1989). Clinical versus actuarial judgment. *Science, 243*, 1668-1674.

Ebbesen, E. B., & Konecni, V. J. (1982). An analysis of the bail system. In V. J. Konecni & E. B. Ebbesen (Eds.), *The criminal justice system: A social-psychological analysis.* San Francisco: Freeman.

Ebert, R. J., & Kruse, T. E. (1978). Bootstrapping the security analyst. *Journal of Applied Psychology, 63*, 110-119.

Edwards, W. (1961). Behavioral decision theory. *Annual Review of Psychology, 12*, 473-498.

Einhorn, H. J. (1972). Expert measurement and mechanical combination. *Organizational Behavior and Human Performance, 7*, 86-106.

Einhorn, H. J. (1980). Learning from experience and suboptimal rules in decision making. In T. Wallsten (Ed.), *Cognitive processes in choice and decision behavior.* Hillsdale, NJ: Lawrence Erlbaum.

Einhorn, H. J., & Hogarth, R. M. (1975). Unit weighting schemes for decision making. *Organizational Behavior and Human Performance, 13*, 171-192.

Einhorn, H. J., & Hogarth, R. M. (1981). Behavioral decision theory: Processes of judgment and choice. *Annual Review of Psychology, 32*, 53-88.

Einhorn, H. J., Kleinmuntz, D. N., & Kleinmuntz, B. (1979). Linear regression and process-tracing models of judgment. *Psychological Review, 86*, 465-485.

Elstein, A. S., & Bordage, G. (1979). Psychology of clinical reasoning. In G. C. Stone, F. Cohen, & N. E. Alder (Eds.), *Health psychology.* San Francisco: Jossey-Bass.

Engel, J. F., Blackwell, R. D., & Miniard, D. (1986). *Consumer behavior* (5th ed.). Hinsdale, IL: Dryden.

Ericsson, K. A., & Simon, H. A. (1984). *Protocol analysis: Verbal reports as data.* Cambridge: MIT Press.

Fischhoff, B. (1975). Hindsight ≠ foresight: The effect of outcome knowledge on judgement under uncertainty. *Journal of Experimental Psychology: Human Perception and Performance, 1*, 288-299.

Fischhoff, B. (1982). Debiasing. In D. Kahneman, P. Slovic, & A. Tversky (Eds.), *Judgment under uncertainty: Heuristics and biases.* New York: Cambridge University Press.

Gilovich, T., Vallone, R., & Tversky, A. (1985). The hot hand in basketball: On the misperception of random sequences. *Cognitive Psychology, 17*, 295-314.

Goldberg, L. R. (1968). Simple models or simple processes? Some research on clinical judgments. *American Psychologist, 23*, 483-496.

Goldstein, W., & Einhorn, H. (1987). Expression theory and the preference reversal phenomena. *Psychological Review, 94*, 236-254.

Gottfredson, D. M., Wilkins, L. T., & Hoffman, P. B. (1978). *Guidelines for parole and sentencing: A policy control method.* Lexington, MA: Lexington.

Green, P. E. (1984). Hybrid models for conjoint analysis: An expository review. *Journal of Marketing Research, 21*, 155-169.

Green, P. E., Helsen, K., & Shandler, B. (1988). Conjoint internal validity under alternative profile. *Journal of Consumer Research, 15,* 392-397.

Green, P. E., & Wind, Y. (1975). New way to measure consumers' judgment. *Harvard Business Review, 53*, 107-117.

Grether, D. M., & Plott, C. (1979). Economic theory of choice and the preference reversal phenomenon. *American Economic Review, 69*, 623-638.

Grochow, J. M. (1972). A utility theoretic approach to evaluation of a time-sharing system. In W. Frieberger (Ed.), *Statistical computer performance evaluation*. New York: Academic Press.

Grochow, J. M. (1973). On user supplied evaluations of time-shared computer systems. *IEEE Transactions on Systems, Man and Cybernetics*, SMC-3, 204-205.

Grofman, B., & Scarrow, H. (1980). Mathematics, social science, and the law. In M. J. Saks & C. H. Baron (Eds.), *The use/nonuse/misuse of applied social research in the courts*. Cambridge, MA: Abt.

Hagarty, M. R., & Aaker, D. A. (1984). A normative model of consumer information. *Marketing Science, 3*, 227-246.

Hammond, K. R., Stewart, T. R., Brehmer, B., & Steinmann, D. O. (1975). Social-judgment theory. In M. F. Kaplan & S. Schwartz (Eds.), *Human judgment and decision processes*. New York: Academic Press.

Hammond, K. R., McClelland, G. H., & Mumpower, J. (1980). *Human judgment and decision making: Theories, methods, and procedures*. New York: Praeger.

Hastie, R., Penrod, S. D., & Pennington, N. (1983). *Inside the jury*. Cambridge, MA: Harvard University Press.

Hoffman, P. J. (1960). The paramorphic representation of clinical judgment. *Psychological Bulletin, 57*, 116-131.

Hoffman, P. J., Slovic, P., & Rorer, L. G. (1968). An analysis-of-variance model for the assessment of configural cue utilization in clinical judgment. *Psychological Bulletin, 69*, 338-349.

Hoffman, L. R. (1979). *The group problem solving process*. New York: Praeger.

Hogarth, R. (1981). Beyond discrete biases: Functional and dysfunctional aspects of judgmental heuristics. *Psychological Bulletin, 90*, 197-217.

Hogarth, R. (1987). *Judgment and choice* (2nd ed). New York: John Wiley.

Huber, G. P. (1980). *Managerial decision making*. Glenview, IL: Scott Foresman.

Humphreys, P., & Berkeley, D. (1983). Problem structuring calculi and levels of knowledge representation in decision making. In R. W. Scholz (Ed.), *Decision making under uncertainty*. New York: North Holland.

Isenberg, D. (1984). How senior managers think. *Harvard Business Review*, November-December, 80-90.

Isenberg, D. J. (1987). Inside the mind of the senior manager. In D. Perkins, J. Lochhead, & J. Bishop (Eds.), *Thinking*. Hillsdale, NJ: Lawrence Erlbaum.

Jacoby, J., Jaccard, J., Kuss, A., Troutman, T., & Mazursky, A. (1985). *New directions in behavioral process research*. New York: New York University Press.

Janis, I. L. (1982). *Groupthink* (2nd ed.). Boston: Houghton Mifflin.

Johnson, E. J. (1988). Expertise and judgment under uncertainty: Performance and process. In M. T. H. Chi, R. Glaser, & M. J. Farr (Eds.), *The nature of expertise*. Hillsdale, NJ: Lawrence Erlbaum.

Johnson, E. J., & Meyer, R. (1984). Compensating choice models of noncompensatory processes: The effect of varying context. *Journal of Consumer Research, 11*, 528-541.

Johnson, E. J., Meyer, R. J., & Ghose, S. (1989). When choice models fail: Compensatory representations in negatively-correlated environments. *Journal of Marketing Research, 26*, 255-270.

Johnson, E. J., & Payne, J. W. (1985). Effort and accuracy in choice. *Management Science 31*, 395-414.

Johnson, E. J., & Russo, J. E. (1984). Product familiarity and learning new information. *Journal of Consumer Research, 11*, 542-550.

Johnson, E. J., & Schkade, D. A. (1989). Bias in utility assessment: Further evidence and explanations. *Management Science, 35*, 406-424.

Kahneman, D., Slovic, P., & Tversky, A. (Eds.) (1982). *Judgment under uncertainty: Heuristics and biases.* New York: Cambridge University Press.

Kahneman, D., & Tversky, A. (1972). Subjective probability: A judgment of representativeness. *Cognitive Psychology, 3*, 430-454.

Kahneman, D., & Tversky, A. (1979). Prospect theory: An analysis of decision under risk. *Econometrica, 47*, 263-291.

Keen, P. G., & Scott-Morton, M. S. (1978). *Decision support systems: An organizational perspective.* Reading, MA: Addison-Wesley.

Keeney, R. L., & Raiffa, H. (1976). *Decision with multiple objectives: Preferences and value tradeoffs.* New York: John Wiley.

Kiesler, S., Siegel J., & McGuire, T. W. (1984). Social psychological aspects of computer-mediated communication. *American Psychologist, 39*, 1123-1134.

Kidder, L. H., & Judd, C. M. (1986). *Research methods in social relations* (5th ed.). New York: Holt, Rinehart, & Winston.

Kleinmuntz, D. N. (1985). Cognitive heuristics and feedback in a dynamic decision environment. *Management Science, 31*, 680-702.

Konecni, V. J., & Ebbesen, E. B. (1979). External validity of research in legal psychology. *Law and Human Behavior, 3*, 39-70.

Konecni, V. J., & Ebbesen, E. B. (1982). An analysis of the sentencing system. In V. J. Konecni & E. B. Ebbesen (Eds.), *The criminal justice system: A social-psychological analysis.* San Francisco: W. H. Freeman.

Lacey, R. (1986). *Ford—The man and the machine.* Boston: Little, Brown.

Lamm, H., & Myers, D. G. (1978). Group induced polarization of attitudes and behavior. In L. Berkowitz (Ed.), *Advances in experimental social psychology, Vol. 11.* New York: Academic Press.

Laughlin, P. R., & Ellis, A. L. (1986). Demonstrability and social combination processes on mathematical intellective tasks. *Journal of Experimental Social Psychology, 22*, 177-189.

Levine, M. (1980). Investigative reporting as a research method: An analysis of Bernstein and Woodward's *All the President's Men. American Psychologist, 35*, 626-638.

Lichtenstein, S., & Slovic, P. (1971). Reversal of preferences between bids and choices in gambling decisions. *Journal of Experimental Psychology, 89*, 46-55.

Lichtenstein, S., & Slovic, P. (1973). Response-induced reversals of preferences in gambling: An extended replication in Las Vegas. *Journal of Experimental Psychology, 101*, 16-20.

Loftus, E. F. (1975). Leading questions and the eyewitness report. *Cognitive Psychology, 7*, 560-572.

Loftus, E. F., & Palmer, J. C. (1984). Reconstruction of automobile destruction: An example of the interaction between language and memory. *Journal of Verbal Learning and Verbal Behavior, 16*, 585-589.

Lord, C., Ross, L., & Lepper, M. R. (1979). Biased assimilation and attitude polarization: The effects of prior theories on subsequently considered evidence. *Journal of Personality and Social Psychology, 37*, 2098-2110.

Lundberg, C. C. (1976). Hypothesis creation in organizational behavior research. *Academy of Management Review, 2*, 5-12.

March, J. G., & Shapira, Z. (1982). Behavioral decision theory and organizational decision theory. In G. R. Ungson & D. N. Braunstein (Eds.), *Decision making: An interdisciplinary inquiry*. Boston: Kent.

March, J. G., & Simon, H. A. (1958). *Organizations*. New York: John Wiley.

Martin, J. (1982). A garbage can model of the research process. In J. E. McGrath, J. Martin, & R. A. Kulka (Eds.), *Judgment calls in research*. Beverly Hills, CA: Sage.

McGrath, J. E. (1982). Dilemmatics: The study of research choices and dilemmas. In J. E. McGrath, J. Martin, & R. A. Kulka (Eds.), *Judgment calls in research*. Beverly Hills, CA: Sage.

Mintzberg, H., Raisinghani, D., & Theoret, A. (1976). The structure of "unstructured" decision processes. *Administrative Science Quarterly, 21*, 246-275.

National Research Council. (1982). *Outlook for science and technology: The next five years*. San Francisco: W. H. Freeman.

Natsoulas, T. (1970). Concerning introspective "knowledge." *Psychological Bulletin, 73*(2), 89-111.

Neter, J., Wasserman, W., & Kuntner, M. H. (1985). *Applied linear statistical models: Regression, analysis of variance, and experimental designs* (2nd ed.). Homewood, IL: Irwin.

Newell, A., & Simon, H. A. (1972). *Human problem solving*. Englewood Cliffs, NJ: Prentice-Hall.

Newman, J. R. (1977). Differential weighting in multiattribute utility measurement: Where it should and where it does make a difference. *Organizational Behavior and Human Performance, 20*, 312-325.

Nisbett, R. E., & Bellows, N. (1977). Verbal reports about causal influences on social judgments: Private access versus public theories. *Journal of Personality and Social Psychology, 35*, 613-624.

Nisbett, R. E., & Ross, L. (1980). *Human inference: Strategies and shortcomings of social judgment*. Englewood Cliffs, NJ: Prentice-Hall.

Nisbett, R. E., & Schachter, S. (1966). Cognitive manipulation of pain. *Journal of Experimental Social Psychology, 2*, 227-236.

Nisbett, R. E., & Wilson, T. D. (1977). Telling more than we can know: Verbal reports on mental processes. *Psychological Review, 84*, 231-259.

Nixon, R. M. (1962). *Six crises*. Garden City, NY: Doubleday.

Onken, J., Hastie, R., & Revelle, W. (1985). Individual differences in the use of simplification strategies in a complex decision-making task. *Journal of Experimental Psychology: Human Perception and Performance, 11*, 14-27.

Parry, H. J., & Crossley, H. M. (1950). Validity of responses to survey questions. *Public Opinion Quarterly, 14*, 61-80.

Payne, J. W. (1976). Task complexity and contingent processing in decision making: An information search and protocol analysis. *Organizational Behavior and Human Performance, 16*, 366-387.

Payne, J. W. (1982). Contingent decision behavior. *Psychological Bulletin, 92*, 382-403.

Payne, J. W., & Braunstein, M. L. (1971). Preferences among gambles with equal underlying distributions. *Journal of Experimental Psychology, 87*, 13-18.

Payne, J. W., & Braunstein, M. L. (1978). Risky choice: An examination of information acquisition behavior. *Memory and Cognition, 5*, 554-561.

Payne, J. W., Braunstein, M. L., & Carroll, J. S. (1978). Exploring pre-decisional behavior: An alternative approach to decision research. *Organizational Behavior and Human Performance, 22*, 17-34.

Petty, R. E., & Cacioppo, J. T. (1981). *Attitudes and persuasion: Classic and contemporary approaches.* Dubuque, IA: Brown.

Powell, W. W. (1985). *Getting into print: The decision-making process in scholarly publishing.* Chicago: University of Chicago Press.

Ravindar, H. V., Kleinmuntz, D. N., & Dyer, J. S. (1988). The reliability of subjective probabilities obtained through decomposition. *Management Science, 34*, 186-199.

Rosenbaum, D., Baumer, T., Bickman, L., Kudel, M., Carroll, J. S., & Perkowitz, W. (1979). *Phase I assessment of shoplifting and employee theft program: Field feasibility assessment of new measurement strategies.* Report to the National Institute of Law Enforcement and Criminal Justice, Law Enforcement Assistance Administration, Department of Justice, Washington, DC.

Russo, J. E. (1978). Eye fixations can save the world: A critical evaluation and a comparison between eye fixations and other information processing methodologies. In H. Hunt. (Ed.), *Advances in consumer research* (Vol. V). Ann Arbor, MI: Association for Consumer Research.

Russo, J. E., & Dosher, B. A. (1983). Strategies for multiattribute binary choice. *Journal of Experimental Psychology: Learning, Memory & Cognition, 4*, 676-696.

Russo, J. E., Johnson, E. J., & Stephens, D. L. (1989). The validity of verbal protocols. *Memory and Cognition, 17*, 759-769.

Schkade, D. A., & Johnson, E. J. (1989). Cognitive processes in preference reversals. *Organizational Behavior and Human Decision Processes, 44*, 203-231.

Shanteau, J., & Nagy, G. (1976). Decisions made about other people: A human judgment analysis of dating choice. In J. S. Carroll & J. W. Payne (Eds.), *Cognition and social behavior.* Hillsdale, NJ: Lawrence Erlbaum.

Sheppard, B. H., Harwick, J., & Warshaw, P. R. (1988). The theory of reasoned action: A meta-analysis of past research with recommendations for modifications and future research. *Journal of Consumer Research, 15*.

Shortliffe, R. H., & Buchanan, B. G. (1984). *Rule based expert systems: The MYCIN experience of the Stanford Heuristic Programming Project.* Reading, MA: Addison-Wesley.

Simon, H. A. (1976). *Administrative behavior* (3rd ed.). New York: Free Press.

Simon, H. A., Smithburg, D. W., & Thompson, V. A. (1950). *Public administration* (1st ed.). New York: Knopf.

Slovic, P. (1969). Analyzing the expert judge: A descriptive study of a stockbroker's decision process. *Journal of Applied Psychology, 53*, 255-263.

Slovic, P., & Lichtenstein, S. (1968). Relative importance of probabilities and payoffs in risk taking. *Journal of Experimental Psychology Monograph, 78*, (3, Pt. 2).

Smith, E. R., & Miller, F. S. (1978). Limits on perception of cognitive processes: A reply to Nisbett and Wilson. *Psychological Review, 85*, 355-362.

Stasser, G. (1988). Computer simulation as a research tool: The DISCUSS model of group decision making. *Journal of Experimental Social Psychology, 24*, 393-422.

Staw, B. (1980). Rationality and justification in organizational life. In B. Staw & L. Cummings (Eds.), *Research in organizational behavior* (Vol. 2, pp. 45-80). New York: JAI Press.

Steiner, I. D. (1972). *Group process and productivity.* New York: Academic Press.

Sterman, J. D. (1987). Misperceptions of feedback in dynamic decision making. *Organizational Behavior and Human Decision Processes, 43,* 301-335.

Sudman, S., & Bradburn, N. (1982). *Asking questions: A practical guide to questionnaire design.* San Francisco: Jossey-Bass.

Svenson, O. (1979). Process descriptions of decision making. *Organizational Behavior and Human Performance, 23,* 86-112.

Thaler, R. (1980). Toward a positive theory of consumer choice. *Journal of Economic Behavior and Organization, 1,* 39-60.

Thaler, R. (1985). Mental accounting and consumer choice. *Marketing Science, 4,* 199-214.

Tversky, A. (1972). Elimination by aspects: A theory of choice. *Psychological Review, 79,* 281-299.

Tversky, A., & Kahneman, D. (1974). Judgment under uncertainty: Heuristics and biases. *Science, 185,* 1124-1131.

Tversky, A., & Kahneman, D. (1981). The framing of decisions and the psychology of choice. *Science, 211,* 453-463.

Tversky, A., Sattath, S., & Slovic, P. (1988). Contingent weighting in judgment and choice. *Psychological Review, 95,* 371-384.

Vinokur, A., & Burnstein, E. (1974). The effects of partially shared persuasive arguments on group-induced shifts: A group-problem-solving approach. *Journal of Personality and Social Psychology, 29,* 305-315.

von Neumann, J., & Morgenstern, D. (1944). *Theory of games and economic behavior.* New York: John Wiley.

von Winterfeldt, D., & Edwards, W. (1986). *Decision analysis and behavioral research.* Cambridge: Cambridge University Press.

Weaver, F. M., & Carroll, J. S. (1985). Crime perceptions in a natural setting by expert and novice shoplifters. *Social Psychology Quarterly, 48,* 349-359.

Wilkie, W. L., & Pessimier, E. A. (1973). Issues in marketing's use of multi-attribute attitude models. *Journal of Marketing Research, 10,* 428-441.

Wright, W. F. (1979). Properties of judgment models in a financial setting. *Organizational Behavior and Human Performance, 23,* 73-85.

Yin, R. K. (1989). *Case study research: Design and methods* (2nd ed.). Beverly Hills, CA: Sage.

Index

About the Authors

John S. Carroll is Professor of Behavioral and Policy Sciences at the MIT. Sloan School of Management, where he teaches courses on decision making, organizational behavior, and behavioral research methods. He was formerly Assistant Professor of Psychology at Carnegie-Mellon University from 1973 to 1978, Associate Professor of Psychology at Loyola University of Chicago from 1978 to 1983, and Visiting Associate Professor of Behavioral Science at the Graduate School of Business of the University of Chicago from 1981 to 1982.

His research focuses on individual and group decision making in organizational and legal settings. Current projects include studies of individual income tax decision making, problem solving in negotiation contexts, and the organization and management of nuclear power plants. He has published three books, most recently *Applied Social Psychology and Organizational Settings,* and has authored numerous journal articles. He is a member of several editorial boards as well as a past member of the National Science Foundation Law and Social Sciences Review Panel.

Dr. Carroll received his BS in Physics from MIT in 1970 and his Ph.D. in Social Psychology from the Department of Psychology and Social Relations at Harvard in 1973. In 1981, he was elected a Fellow of the American Psychological Association.

Eric J. Johnson is Associate Professor of Marketing and Decision Science at the Wharton School of the University of Pennsylvania. After graduation from Rutgers University, he received his MS and Ph.D. in Psychology from Carnegie-Mellon University, and was a National Science Foundation postdoctoral fellow at Stanford. He previously has taught at Carnegie-Mellon, the Sloan School at MIT, and Chulalongkorn University in Bangkok.

His principal research interests include consumer and managerial decision making and the cognitive processes underlying simple judgments and choice. His publications have appeared in the *Journal of Personality and Social Psychology, Journal of Consumer Research, Journal of Marketing Research, Management Science, Organizational Behavior and Human Decision Processes,* and the *Journal of Experimental Psychology.*

137

Professor Johnson serves on the editorial boards of several journals and is currently pursuing the application of behavioral decision research to insurance decision making and to competitive games.

NOTES

NOTES

NOTES

NOTES

NOTES

NOTES